Polyvagal Theory

The Secrets Behind the Rhythm of Regulation

(Learn How Is Polyvagal Theory a Way Out to Reduce Mental Stress)

Tomas Barnes

Published By **Andrew Zen**

Tomas Barnes

All Rights Reserved

Polyvagal Theory: The Secrets Behind the Rhythm of Regulation (Learn How Is Polyvagal Theory a Way Out to Reduce Mental Stress)

ISBN 978-1-77485-655-0

No part of this guidebook shall be reproduced in any form without permission in writing from the publisher except in the case of brief quotations embodied in critical articles or reviews.

Legal & Disclaimer

The information contained in this ebook is not designed to replace or take the place of any form of medicine or professional medical advice. The information in this ebook has been provided for educational & entertainment purposes only.

The information contained in this book has been compiled from sources deemed reliable, and it is accurate to the best of the Author's knowledge; however, the Author cannot guarantee its accuracy and validity and cannot be held liable for any errors or omissions. Changes are periodically made to this book. You must consult your doctor or get professional medical advice before using any of the suggested remedies, techniques, or information in this book.

Upon using the information contained in this book, you agree to hold harmless the Author from and against any damages, costs, and expenses, including any legal fees potentially resulting from the application of any of the information provided by this guide. This disclaimer applies to any damages or injury caused by the use and application, whether directly or indirectly, of any advice or information presented, whether for breach of contract, tort, negligence, personal injury, criminal intent, or under any other cause of action.

You agree to accept all risks of using the information presented inside this book. You need to consult a professional medical practitioner in order to ensure you are both able and healthy enough to participate in this program.

Table Of Contents

Chapter 1: The Basics Of The Autonomic Nervous Système And Vagus Nerve 1

Chapter 2: Polyvagal Theory & The Vagus Nerve 21

Chapter 3: The Effects Of Vagal Tone On Our Nervous System 30

Chapter 4: Social Engagement And Defensive Behaviour 45

Chapter 5: Children, Emotional Resulation And Polyvagal Thory 65

Chapter 6: Trauma, The Flaw Of The System 80

Chapter 7: Connecting With Your Higherself... 90

Chapter 8: Functions Of Vagus Nerve .. 101

Chapter 9: Clinical Utilizations Of The Polyvagal Hypothesis 120

Chapter 10: Parasympathetic System .. 143

Chapter 11: Borderline Personality Disorder And Emotion Regulation 152

Chapter 12: Vagus Nerve Yoga 164

Conclusion 181

Chapter 1: The Basics Of The Autonomic Nervous Système And Vagus Nerve

The Anatomical Structure

This section will discuss the anatomy and functions of the vagus neuron.

The vagus, also known by the tenth brain stem CN or nerve number X, is a long nerve. It originates within the human brain stem. It then stretches down to the neck and into your chest.

The motor is a combination of sensory and motor information. It supplies innervation through the center to major blood vessels.

Although there are generally two vagus brains (the left as well as the right), doctors tend to refer to them both collectively under the name vagus nerve.

The vagus nervous can control the muscles of the throat and voicebox. It is vital in controlling the heartbeat and maintaining a healthy gastrointestinal tract. The inner organs on the brain also provide sensory info to the vagus neurons.

Feature of Vagus Nerve

The vagus nervous is perhaps the most important. It distributes parasympathetic fibrils to the main organs of your body (the abdomen, chest or head), and is responsible for the distribution of parasympathetic energy.

The vagus nervous is susceptible to the development of a cough reflex. If the ear is stimulated, it stimulates the peristalsis mechanism in the digestive tract. This controls the heart rate and blood pressure as well as controlling the vascular tone.

The Vasovagal Reflex

Unexpected stimulations of the vagus nerve can produce what's known to be a "vasovagal effect," which results in an unexpected drop in the blood pressure and a slower heart beat.

This reflex could be triggered by gastrointestinal illness, or possibly in response to fear, pain, or tension unexpectedly.

Vasovagal reactions can be very dangerous for many people. In addition to blood pressure changes and pulse rate changes that can lead to loss consciousness, there is also a condition called "vasovagal Syncope". Certain medical conditions, particularly dysautonomy may also experience excessive vagus nervous activation.

Description Sensory. Innervates external auditory and meat skins, as well as the internal laryngopharynx surfaces and laryngopharynx. Provides abdominal tactile feeling and heart stimulation.

Special Sensory. Provides an epiglottis- and tongue root senses.

Motor: Provides motor stimulation for most pharynxs, palates and larynx muscles.

Parasympathy. Innervates the trachea's smooth muscle, bronchis, and digestive tract. It also controls heart rhythm.

The vagus nerve, which runs from head-to-abdomen, has the longest series (if any) of cranial neuros. Latin' vagary' means wandering. It is sometimes called wandering brain.

In Head

The brainstem is the source of the vagus and medulla. It also exits into the cranium along with accessory nerves CN IX and XI (respectively) and glossopharyngeal over the jugularforamen.

The cranium contains the uricular tree. This produces sensation in the external auditory and external ears.

The vagus is a nerve that runs through the carotid skin, and flows inferiorly with the inner carotid artery and jugular vein. At the base, the pathways of the right and left neck nerves are different: The right vagus is located before the subclavic blood vessel and the sternoclavicular joint.

The left vagus nerve moves inferiorly into the thorax between the left popular carotid and left subclavic arteries, post-sternoclavicular joint.

There are many branches that grow in the neck.

Motor innervation to the soft palate muscles and pharynx can be provided by the pharyngeal branch.

Superior laryngeal and cricothyroid nerves split into outside and inside branches. The laryngeal innervates cricothyroid's muscle. The internal laryngeal gives tactile innervation of the laryngopharynx, and the upper larynx.

Recurrent laryngeal nervous (only on the right).-Hassles under the right supraclavic artery and then ascends to larynx. Innervates most of larynx's intrinsic muscle.

The posterior vagal tree in the thorax is formed with the right vagus and the anterior vagal tree with the left. The vagal trunks branches are responsible for the formation of an oesophageal complexus. This connects to the smooth muscle at the oesophagus.

Two branches are also visible in the thorax.

Cardiac Branch-- These innervates regulate heartbeat and give the organ visceral sensation.

The abdominal vagal trunks attach to the diaphragm through the diaphragm-opening oesophageal hiatus.

The vagal trunks are found in the abdomen. They split into branches, which supply the oesophagus (up until the splenic Flexure), intestine, and small and larger bowel.

Sensory functions The Vagus nerve sensor system has both visceral and somatic components.

Somatic refers the skin and muscle sensation. This is achieved by the auricular, or inner auditory nerve.

Viscera feeling comes from the body's organs. Vagus nerve innervates, laryngopharynx through the laryngeal neural nerve.

Superior larynx dimension (above the vocal folds) - via the laryngeal neuro.

Heart-Through cardiac nerve branches.

Gastrointestinal tract (upto splenic extension)-through the vagus nerve terminal branches.

The vagus neuron also plays a role in taste sensation. This nerve contains the epiglottis root fibrous and the afferent tooth.

This should be understood in conjunction with the sensation that the glossopharyngeal nerve provides, which is a sensation of taste for 1/3 of the posterior tongue.

Motor functions

The vagus neural communicates all muscles related to the pharynx. These muscles control swallowing and phoning.

Pharynx Most of the pharyngeal and pharyngeal musculatures are also innervated through the vagus neural's pharyngeal branches.

Salpingopharyngeus as well as Palatopharyngeus. A glossopharyngeal neuro innervates a second pharyngeal muscle, the stylopharyngeal.

Larynx Innervation occurs through the recurrent laryngeal neural nerve and superior laryngeal inner branch.

Recurrent laryngeal nerve symptoms are as follows:

Lateral Crico-arytenoid

Thyro-arytenoid

Oblique and transversely distributed arytenoids

Posterior posterior-cricoarytenoid

Vocalis Inner laryngeal Nerve: Cricothyroid Other Muscles The vagus nerve interferes frequently with the palatoglossus, the tongue and the weakest palate muscles.

The vagus neuro is the main parasympathetic neural outflow from the digestive organs and to the heart. It can be found in the abdomen, thorax, and stomach.

Core cardiac branches originate in the thorax, conveying parasympathetic innervation straight to the heart'satrio-ventricular and sino-atrial nodes

Both divisions cause a decline in heart rate. They are constantly active and produce 60-80 beats an hour. The heart rate could be as high as 100 beats/minute, if the vagus nervous were to be severed.

Gastrointestinal systems The vagus neuron provides parasympathetic invation to most abdominal and other organs. It sends branches into the oesophagus (to the stomach), most intestinal tract and the large colon's Splenic Flexure.

Vagus nerve function is stimulate glandular secretions in those organs and smooth muscular contraction. The vagus nervous stimulates acid secretion and increases stomach emptying.

The Vagus nerve (and Nervous System)

The vagus nervous's most important feature is the Afferent. It brings information on the human body about the internal organs.

It means that the most important sources of sensory data on the brain are the organs within it. The intestine is the highest-reaching organ in the sensory body and has the potential to be particularly important.

The vagus is an antagonist of both the sympathetic nervous and efferent systems. It has been studied in the past. Parasympathetic efferents can be obtained from most organs by the splanchnic nerves that include the vagus and sympathetic nerves.

The parasympathetic nerve system and the sympathetic nervous system are responsible for any regulation of vegetative functions by acting in opposite directions. The parasympathetic innervation is responsible for dilation of blood vessels, bronchioles, and stimulation of salivary glands.

The sympathetic innervation however, causes blood vessel contraction, bronchiol dislation, increased heartbeat, and constriction or the intestinal and urinary sphincters. Parasympathetic nerve system activation in the gastrointestinal tract increases glandular production and bowel movement.

Because of this, the sympathetic function results in a decrease blood circulation, intestinal activity to the stomach and an increase in blood pumping.

The ENS comes from neural crest cells that are predominantly vagal eman. It is composed of a nerve plexus located in the intestinal walls. This nerve plexus stretches from esophagus into the anus, and runs throughout the entire gastrointestinal track. It is estimated that between 100 and 500,000,000 neurons make up the human ENS.

This is the location with the greatest concentration of nerves cells. It is similar to a brain in terms of chemical coding function and structure. Therefore, it is sometimes called the intestinal second mind or brain.

It consists of two submucosal-ganglionated plexuses. This controls gastrointestinal blood circulation and regulates epithelial capacity and secretion.

The ENS acts like an intestinal barrier and regulates essential enteric activities such as immune reaction, nutrient detect, motility microvascular blood circulation and water, ion and bioactive peptide epithelial secretion.

There is certainly interaction between ENS and vagal nerves in general. Cholinergic activation using nicotinic receptors is the primary transmitter. A bidirectional flow of information occurs when the ENS and vagal nerves contact each other.

The ENS can, however, function in isolation of vagal control in the large intestines.

We control the activity, motility, and fluxes in substances of muscles and mucosal blood. ENS neurons can also interact with the cells in the immune system of the adaptive or innate body, and even control their roles.

Cell and old damage in the ENS can lead to constipation, problems with evacuation, and incontinence. The loss or destruction of the ENS at the large and the small intestines may be life-threatening (Hirschsprung's Disease; intestinal pseudoobstruction). But, the vagal nerve is not affected at these sites.

Bradycardia sinus activation can also be caused by the right nerve of the vagus. The stimulation for the AV nerve can come from the left vagus, and it is possible to cause a heart block. Valsalva maneuver produces a temporary heart obstruction that can prevent most SVT types.

Medical science has been involved for decades in vagus neural stimulation or blockage because it has many important functions.

Vagotomy, which involves cutting the vagus, was a commonly used treatment for peptic ulcer disease. It is a method to lower the amount of stomach acid. Despite its many negative effects, vagotomy is much less popular today and can be replaced with more effective treatment.

Electronic stimulators (mainly altered ratemakers) are a popular choice today to continuously stimulate the vagus to treat various health problems.

These devices (commonly called VNS devices or vagus-neuro-stimulating device) were commonly used to treat severe epilepsy. It is also used for refractory and severe depression.

VNS devices that are designed to treat other conditions like migraines, tinnitus or fibromyalgia can also be manufactured by companies.

These VNS implementations give hope. VNS will only realize its true potential if solid clinical evidence replaces the uncertainty. The vagus, the principal contributor to parasympathetic neural system, is tenth in cranial nerves from the Medulla Oblongata.

Cell bodies of vagal neuron cells are found in the ambiguous cell nucleus (NA), as well as the vagus lateral motor (DMV). These nuclei supply fibers which are connected to the vagus neural via the cranium via the Jugular Foramen.

At the level of the jugular andamen, the vagus' superior, jugular, ganglion provides the Auriculus with cutaneous branching and internal acoustic meus. A second ganglion (the nodose ganglion) receives visceral tissues sensory innervation.

The cell bodies (or sensory) neurons of an erent (i.e. sensory) neuron travel to this nucleus via the second ganglion. This nucleus relays medulla data to regulate cardiovascular, respiratory, GI function.

The cervical vagus descends in the carotid herath, between the internal jugular and carotid vessels. The subclavian arterial and aortic arch stages are where the recurrent, left- and right-side laryngeal neural nerves contribute to cardiac innervation.

The Vagus Nerve serves as an Intestinal Barrier

Through close junctions, epithelial cells within the intestine create a strict barrier between outside and internal interactions. Close junctions are made of trans membrane proteins like claudins as well as occludins.

In the absence of epithelial membrane integrity and tight junction expression, bacterial translocation can occur across the intestinal mucosa. This could lead to systemic inflammation.

Some studies showed that glial cells activation triggers S-nitrosoglutathione's (GSNO), which releases, increasing the expression and mucosal integrity.

These results have also been confirmed in vivo with intraperitoneal i.p. GNSO injections in inflammatory models.97-100Vagus Neuron and Intestinal Immune Systems: To date, electrical vagus nerve stimulation has been used to treat intractable epilepsy as well as treatment-resistant depression.

Currently VNS was found to have anti-inflammatory e like effects in three clinical studies with patients suffering from Crohn's disease, RA and post-operative ileus.

A functioning VNS or vagus can improve communication between brain and body as well as the operation of your own body.

To increase vagal tone, you can use breathing exercises and cold blasts. If you need further assistance, both you and your doctor can decide to implant a vagus stimulator.

The vagal pathway is a nerve network that connects out from the brain and regulates several bodies within the body, such as the heart and lungs. Modern medicine treats the individual organs in the same way as diseases. Your brain gets a vagus nerve state check from each organ to determine how things work.

It's like a twin lane. The brain does not change if everything goes according to plan. The vagus nerve can be used to signal that an organ is in danger and give your brain more energy. The vagus nervous relays messages from your brain to organs, when your body is ready to move.

Your vaguely nerve needs to function properly in order to ensure nothing is lost. Your vaguely managed ways of controlling things, such as food intakes and hunger hormones or anxiety, are essential for the brain's and organs.

It has many innervation modalities and is functionally different. It is related to the derivatives of fourth and sixth pharyngeal rings.

Chapter 2: Polyvagal Theory & The Vagus Nerve

Before we proceed, we need to examine the Polyvagal Theory. If you want to understand the Polyvagal Theory in its entirety, you will need to be able comprehend how the vagus nervous system and the body interact with it. The nervous system is a complex and interconnected system. We will only briefly discuss the parts. What is important is how the body interacts with the rest of the world. It examines how your body responds to intense stress and how it can keep you alive. We will discuss the theory, and also the anatomy of each vagus nerve.

This chapter will cover all you need to know about the Polyvagal Theory. When you are able to understand the theory, you will be able to apply it in your everyday interactions with others. You will understand the reasons behind your behavior and how it affects others. This will allow you to be more effective in dealing with specific situations.

The Polyvagal Theory

Polyvagal Theory could be simplified to mean understanding the nervous system's response to life-threatening and dangerous situations. It is how your body is trying to keep yourself alive in the present. This is a little too simplified. But it is how your body responds, regulates, and reacts to stress. Polyvagal Theory examines not only your stress response but also how you feel when you are in relaxation.

It examines the fact that you can be in three modes at once. We already know that these are the fight, flight, and freeze modes. The rest, digest, or your relaxation and socializing mode, is basically the third mode. These three modes change based on what is happening around them. The vagus brain is responsible for this. There are several parts to the one vagus brain. These will be discussed later.

The Polyvagal Theory helps to understand how each part of your vagus neuron activates to regulate your own body. The vagus neuron is largely inhibitory. If activated enough it takes control from the sympathetic nerve system (which regulates your fight/flight response), or it stops activating completely, then that fight/flight response can take control. Sometimes, it triggers too many times, triggering a freeze-reaction. When this happens, your body shuts off. We'll be discussing these parts of your vagus nerve in more detail soon.

This is important because you can see exactly why people respond the way that they do. It helps you understand the reasons the world works the way that it does. You can see how each of these emotions work and how they are related. You will be able recognize how your stress will affect you and what you can do to alleviate it.

Four points will be particularly relevant to you based on the Polyvagal Theory.

Trauma, PTSD and Other Psychological Disorders: These are two things that most people don't want to face in their lives. Trauma is inevitable. Most people will experience some type of traumatic event at one time or another. The Polyvagal Theory will allow you to discover how trauma and PTSD can be handled and what it can do you and your family.

Relationships. Once you have mastered the Polyvagal Theory, your ability to recognize how the relationships between you and others will play out will come in handy. The relationship you are in will be apparent to you. You must be in proper vagal activation for people to have meaningful relationships.

Stress on the brain: You'll learn to recognize how extreme stress can damage the body.

When you dissociate, it is like you're completely disconnected from the outside world. We will be looking into this more in detail.

Reading body language. Finally, understanding the Polyvagal Theory will allow you to understand how bodylanguage is actually received thanks to activation and socialization. In this way, you will learn how to support yourself and tap into the inherent ability to read body language. This is a very powerful skill and can help facilitate better, more fluid relationships.

You will eventually be able use this in many different settings in your life. You'll see that prosocial behavior itself is linked to the neuronal autonomic system. It is therefore important that your vagus nerve be in tip-top shape if you want to maintain a healthy social lifestyle. It's only then that you can begin to understand exactly how you need interact with the world around.

Also, you will be able to see how the vagus neural itself is connected to your health. The vagus brain is already regulatory so it will not be surprising that prolonged periods of flight or freeze will have negative consequences for the body. Your body is flooded with stress hormones. These are good times to activate them occasionally but they shouldn't be long-term. The vagus nerve can only be activated if you are able to understand the process.

Anatomy of the Vagus Nerve

This is where we will address the anatomy. You can easily see that your vagus nerve is made up of two distinct structures: your ventral and dorsal. This will allow you to identify and control the different branches of the vagus neuro.

Dorsal vagal compound: This section of the vagus is located at the dorsal muscle nucleus. It is most often unmyelinated. This means that it doesn't usually have the myelin covering that modern neurons have. Myelin sheaths can allow impulses from your brain to travel faster and easier through the neuron. They typically are found on most neurons. They are however absent from the vagus neural branch. This branch, regardless what their classification, is found in almost all vertebrates. This means even frogs, reptiles, and others that are primitive evolutionarily or have remained unchanged for millennia will have this particular nerve. This nerve triggers a basic freeze response. You can think about this: What happens when you scare an animal? It freezes. They usually stop moving entirely because they are afraid. This is an attempt to preserve and regulate the animal's metabolism. Even though mammals have more vagus nerves than their counterparts in mammals, we will soon be discussing these. This section of the vagus is responsible to control the visceral Organs. It controls the areas under the diaphragm. This is because your body does not require you to digest food if you are trying to conserve energy.

Ventral vagal Complex: This is the other component of the vagus neuron that needs to be considered. This particular section was designed to be more recent and was part of the evolution process for mammals. It allows for intelligent, rational responses to all the surrounding world. Instead of defaulting to refusing to acknowledge or freezing completely, it allows you to be more intelligent. When you look at the ventral nerve complex, you see the area where the vagus nerve will control the fight/flight complex. It is the "smart" vagus, so to say. It allows you the ability to visualize what is happening and determine the best response. This usually happens through activating the sympathetic nervous by muting vagal activation. It allows the brain make a decision on whether it wants to fight or flee. But, when the ventral valve complex activates, you will also notice other changes in the body. The ventral vagal activation is when you start to see prosocial behaviors.

The dorsal valgal complex, which is the primitive region of the vagus neuro that triggers your freeze reaction, is therefore the basic area. Your ventral Vagal Complex is responsible for keeping calm when you feel afraid or stressed. Your ventral valve complex can also stop working, allowing for a sympathetic response that could lead to fighting or fleeing. These three systems combine to determine how you are likely to react. This also brings back the importance the vagus brain as an emotional regulator. The vagus nerve is the main factor in determining how an individual responds to the outside world.

Chapter 3: The Effects Of Vagal Tone On Our Nervous System

What does the polyvagal hypothesis have on our neurological system, and what are its implications?

Let's look at this briefly to see how it can have an impact on our health. This chapter will discuss vagal tone.

Prior to the discovery by the Polygala Theory of our bodies, we believed that we had a nervous sistem with two opposing sides. One was parasympathetic, while the other was sympathetic. Both these sides are diametrically opposed and will result in relaxation or stimulation. While they don't fight, their activities may be diametrically opposed. This can lead to confusion.

The Polyvagal Theory focuses on the interplay of three different types nerve system reactions. This is what makes them so important.

The third nervous function acts as a bridge to the parasympathetic or sympathetic nervous systems. This system is also distinct in its involvement in social engagement. The social engagement system makes it easy to address diverse interpersonal interactions.

These two sections help us in life-threatening situations. They assist us in creating various defense mechanisms to help us defend ourselves when in danger.

We all have heard of the fight/flight response. This is normally controlled by the sympathetic nervous system. The other option is the social interaction mechanism to resolve issues. This one requires greater reason and, sometimes, the application if safety and socialization in order to defend yourself.

Both the parasympathetic (and sympathetic) nervous systems are very important components of your nervous system. Polyvagal Theory however shows that both segments of the vagus neuron do relieve the body. However, in different ways. Remember our discussion about the different complexes? The Polyvagal Theory is a different approach to calming down.

The dorsal branch in his neurological system controls your shutdown, free-or–faint, or slowed response. It's mostly responsible for weary muscles lightheadedness, flu-like symptoms, and even lightheadedness. This one can be harmful to your heart or lungs. But it can also impact your digestive tract, and cause problems with your function.

As I mentioned, the ventral, or branch, of the vagus is located just above the diaphragm. It is the one that is more socially connected. It houses the brain as well as the lungs and heart. This is critical because it can help decrease the body's active status. You should be calm if your anxiety is not overwhelming.

What does this control look and feel like?

This can be visualized by picturing yourself riding a horse to the stables. You can continue pulling on the reins or let go so the horse has the ability to maintain its speed. It will also help you to brake when you are required.

Let's suppose you are in control of a horse. Let's assume you have to take him uphill. To overcome the drag caused by climbing uphill you can get your horse to go a little faster. Windy conditions may mean you have to work harder.

What if the speed of the horse causes it to accelerate up, but you don't want him to crash into the fence? You must also keep the horse under control. The Polyvagal Theory works the same. The vagus neuron is important because it helps calm and stimulate the body. Ventral vagus neuro functions in a way which aids in sympathetic activation regulation.

Ventral vagal tone only releases activity in a fraction, but sympathetic activation takes far longer. It takes only a few extra seconds for sympathetic activation to take place because of the chemical interactions that are required in order to regulate your body. Although sympathetic activation takes longer than normal, it can take almost 20 minutes to return you to the stage prior to fight or flight.

Because of this, we have to make changes faster between them. The polyvagal theory basically controls as many as possible.

Here's a second example. Let's assume you have a pet dog and want to take it to a park. You may just want to visit the dog park and look at their pets. Some dogs won't approach you because they fear for their safety. It's easy to dismiss them as "he doesn't care" but they are actually engaging in fight-or flee response.

Some dogs might be begging to play, and they may even bring you their ball. This is their way to show that they want to socialize. This is what you would expect to see in dogs. It's a similar behavior to a yoga downward dog. If a dog gives this signal, it can produce a high degree of arousal and a lot of energy.

However, their joyful energy is much more intense than those of other fight or flight behaviours. These fun energies, along with their playful personalities, are essential components of the social involvement system. If we can experience the world in an easier way, we function better from this social interaction system. Being reassured in your surroundings will reduce anxiety and allow you to relax.

In reality, controlling the neurological system can be difficult. It'd be easier to manage our reactions. We wouldn't even know that we are dependent on this system.

But, traumas and other disorders can alter our vagal tone, and even the neurological system. That is a problem. Let's begin by discussing vagal tone. It's an important aspect of how vagal complexes work together.

What is Vagal Tone and what does it mean for you?

To start, vagal toning refers to how the body reacts to the vagus nervous. Our central nervous systems will respond to different environmental signals via neural input in order to maintain body homeostasis. These environmental cues aid us in determining the best time to respond to various body parts. Stress can disrupt the rhythmic organization these autonomic state's and lead to actions that are not as intended.

Yes, stress can affect the vagus nerve. Vagus nerve irritation can cause a variety of symptoms.

The vital role of the vagus neuro in all these processes, particularly in peripheral nervous system heart rate and respiration rates, can have a major impact on your body's heart beat.

Many people don't realize that vagal tone is adjustable, but only to certain degrees. The respiratory sinus Arrhythmia (or respiratory sinus arrhythmia) is a measurement that basically depicts the parasympathetic nervous activity via heart and how it works.

The RSA is a noninvasive method to monitor our vagal tone. You can use it to watch how the vagus regulates stress response and heart rate. You can actually measure the vagal tone of a person to see how they react to stress.

All of us deal with stress every day. The majority of people are affected by stress at some point in their lives.

Some people might not even be reacting at all to stress. They might react to stress in excess occasionally. Stress is an inevitable part of human life. There are healthy levels and dangerous amounts.

RSA is a very good method, as it will show how much the heart beat changes with breathing. The RSA will display the efferent impact of the vagus neural on the heart or lungs. Studies have been done to prove this.

It will also show how different body components are affected by vagus nerve stimulation. The vagus nerve's inhibitions of its ventricular branch allows for a variety of prosocial, adaptive behaviours. The result is that you can see how the body adapts to social situations and how these actions react under stress.

A higher vagal tone is both desirable and undesirable. A high vagal tone indicates that your actions are being controlled. It is important that it doesn't get outof control. If you feel stressed or overwhelmed, this can cause you to feel anxious. Many people do not have a high vagal tone. Many people have a lower vagal tone than others. This can lead to many issues from mental challenges to illnesses. Reduced vagal tone may cause anxiety and problems with the heart or lungs.

What Can We Learn From Vagal Tone

What can our vagal tone reveal about us? Vagal tone serves as a psychological and medical research tool for better understanding the physiological imprinting that many illnesses have.

This can be applied for a human foetus in order to determine its variability. If the foetus is in a healthy environment, the heart rate will be high and steady. However, when the foetus experiences stress, its heart rate decreases and its vagal tone is decreased.

The vagal influence from your heart has an effect on the dorsal Vagal Control.

The vagal tone determines the health of the heart. Brachycardia, an abnormally low heart rate, may be affected by the vagal tone. The physiological vulnerability affects the heart's state. The onset of this condition is often preceded with a condition called "tachycardia", which is a rapid heartbeat. It is due to the loss or control of vagal function.

Your heart rate will spike if you're in stress or confronted with stressful situations. If you control your vagal tone, and have complete control over your vagus nerve, your heart rate can drop dramatically. This is a sign that you are happy.

This is why the Polyvagal Theory (and vagal tone) can be used as tools to determine our vagus nervous system's general state. The way we respond to the stimuli around us determines whether or no work is needed to improve our vagal tone.

The Polyvagal Theory can provide some insight on the biology and safety hazards we face as well as the interaction of our visceral experience within our bodies with the voices or faces we encounter.

Vagal Tone - The Role of Different Faces

Our vagal tone will be affected by the company we associate. Our vagus nerves are naturally activated by people who have a calm and friendly demeanour. It's the reason we get upset when things become too hard for us to manage.

The body can respond to vagal tonality in a variety ways. There is much to be gained. Learn more about the benefits of vagal Tone.

Many people don't know that the people with whom we are surrounded can affect our vagal tone. High-stimulus environs can make people feel more stressed. For example, if it's a hard day at work, or you're surrounded with people who stress them out, you may feel anxious. This is also why it's possible to feel scared, insecure and unhappy around others.

It's also the reason that it's beneficial to spend time after a stressful event with people who are kind, supportive, and don't make you feel anxious or scared. Your feelings are affected by those people who are important in your life.

Mothers who are comforting to their child's weeping might help them to feel better. Mothers who are too harsh on their children may cause a whole host of problems. People who surround themselves with pleasant and calm people can feel more secure and at ease. People who are unkind to them will make them miserable.

When you surround yourself with people who are kind to you, you'll feel more secure and tranquil. People find it difficult to accept being rejected or ignored. However, polyvagal theory can make it worse and lead to mental illness and wrath. If we don't invest in developing these social skills, we'll be forced to resort to the fight or flight mode which will result in hibernation. This theory sheds light onto the significance of social behaviors and the trauma that supports them.

Chapter 4 will provide more information about trauma and the role of the vagus nervous system in your experience. Regardless of whether your trauma is PTSD, you will need to have different methods to focus and repair your body. Understanding your body's system will prove to be very useful. There is much happening now that will undoubtedly benefit you.

The vagus nervous is a strong nerve. Knowing your Polyvagal Theory can help you understand this nerve. This can assist us in managing stressful situations and will help us grow and improve our lives.

This nerve can be extremely powerful. We all know it exists and should stimulate it. What is the effect of this stimulation on the entire body? What can you learn from this? With all that information in mind and everything going on you can see the extent of the polyvagal hypothesis as well the vagus neuron. We will explore this anatomy in more detail, as well as the potential effects on people.

Chapter 4: Social Engagement And Defensive Behaviour

Depending on the extent of the hazards that exist in the world, social commitments and defensive methods can be either flexible or inappropriate. From a clinical standpoint, the defining characteristics of psychopathology include either failure to repress guard mechanisms in a sheltered environment or inability of individuals to initiate protection system in an unsafe area. Only in a protected context is it appropriate and versatile to hinder barriers and exhibit positive social commitment. Broken neuroception, or an incorrect evaluation about the wellbeing and peril of a scenario, may increase the maladaptive physiological response and the declaration of protective practices in relation to mental disorders. Neuroception still recognizes opportunity precisely when children are created.

Children's intellectual familiarity in hazard coordinates "gut reactions" to risk.

Our metabolic needs alter when our nervous sistem recognizes security. Stress reactions that are related with fight and flight, for example, increments in pulse and cortisol intervened by the thoughtful nervous system and hypothalamic-pituitary-adrenal pivot--are hosed. As well, neuroception of wellbeing protects us in physiological states such a massive drop in circulatory strain, pulse, fainting and apnea. These are all signs that can be used to support "freezing" as well as "shutdown".

How does your nervous system detect when the earth has become dangerous or sheltered? What neural systems evaluate hazard in the natural world? Functional attractive reverberation image imaging has recently identified neural structures that help to detect hazard. Some regions of our minds are capable of identifying and assessing highlights. This includes facial and body development as well as vocalizations that enhance our sense of wellbeing and dependability. Scientists identified a specific region of the cortex that reacts when we hear well-known voices and natural faces. The cortex' worldly flap is responsible for this process of identifying reliable individuals and assessing the goals of others dependent upon "organic advancements" of face or appendages. If neuroception classifies an individual's status as "sheltered", then a neural circuit effectively restricts territories of mind that are used to distinguish between the guarded strategies of freeze, fight, and flight. Changes in the organic processes that we see could shift neuroception from "safety" into "perilous." When this happens, the neural structures that control prosocial conduct and those related to protective techniques become activated.

At that point, the dynamic hindrance that governs guard methodologies in the cerebrum territories gives the opportunity for social conduct to occur immediately at the sight and eye of a sheltered person. The presence of a companion, or guardian, would suppress the neural circuits within the mind that regulate cautious techniques. In this way, it becomes possible to make close physical contact with others and to engage in social commitments. The mind circuits that are designed to protect you from danger can also be activated in times of crisis. Social methods are dealt with by forceful behavior or withdrawal.

Fearless immobilization

As we have seen, people have three head protection methodologies--fight, flight, and freeze. Although we have a good understanding of fight and flight strategies, we tend to forget about immobilization. This technique was first taught to vertebrates as "death pretending". As humans, we observe a conduct shutdown. Sometimes, this is joined by extremely fragile muscle tone. We also monitor physiological changes. Our pulse and breathing slow down, while our circulatory strain drops.

One of the oldest safeguards for animals is freezing or immobilization. Repressing the development of our animals reduces our appetite and our need for food, and it increases our pain edge. Despite being frozen, warm blooded creatures can still remain in place for basic prosocial actions, including childbirth, origination, and nursing. When a baby is nurtured by a mother, she must restrict her growth. Functionally immobilized occurs when a child's grasp is made. Regenerative practices also include some form of immobilization. Immunization with dread may cause dangerous physiological changes. Through the process of developing, neural circuits in our minds that were initially associated wit freezing practices were modified to satisfy personal social requirements. These mind structures were eventually able to recognize a neuropeptide, oxytocin. During nursing and birth, oxytocin gets released. It is also released during social bonding exercises. When we feel our condition has been protected, oxytocin is released to allow us to take comfort in the grasp. However, oxytocin is not released when our nervous system detects that someone is dangerous.

Social Engagement: The Preamble For A Social Bond

To form a bond with others, it is essential to stop resistance systems. A person should be open to the possibility of being genuinely close to another. This is true whether it's a mother and her baby creating a relationship or two adults forming a bond. There are many differences in the contexts where mother-newborn infant connection takes place and the social obligations for conceptive accomplices.

They are already set up. Consider versatility. Because of juvenile neural advance, the baby's movement ability is restricted. It is likely that two grown-ups will have similar conduct collections, which could lead to them becoming conceptive partners.

The making of social bonds depends on deliberate engine techniques. At that point, the human infant will be greatly burdened. The neural guidance of the spinal engines pathways is young at the hour of birth. It takes quite a while for it to mature completely. Social commitment does require that we are able to manage our body and appendages. Willful trunk development (i.e., corticospinal neural pathways) and willful appendage require neural pathways connecting brainstem to spinal nerves. Social commitment is more dependent on our ability manage the muscles that make up our heads and bodies. These pathways connect the cortex to the brainstem (corticobulbar routes). These are the muscles which give our face a personality and allow us to use our heads to send signals, to put pitch into voices, to control our eyes, and to distinguish human voices from foundation sounds. The muscles controlling the storage compartment, appendages and muscles of the spine are directed by corticospinal channels to spinal nerves. The muscles controlling the facial and head muscles are managed by corticobulbar routes to cranial and cranial nerves. The neural pathways to these nerves (i.e. cortex) are adequately myelinated in childbirth. This allows newborns to flag guardians by vocalizing or smiling; corticobulbar pathways to cranial nerves manage the muscles of the face and head.

The neural guideline of the facial muscles and the head influences how an individual sees the commitment patterns of others. Particularly, this neural line can help to reduce social seperation by allowing people (counting newborn children):

*Make eye contact with your eye connection

*vocalize with an engaging rhythm and intonation

*display unforeseen exterior appearances;

*Modulate the center-ear muscles to seperate the human voice and foundation sound more effectively

You may also notice a decrease in muscle tone, which is caused by a neuroception (or a life risk) in an external condition (e.g. hazardous individuals or circumstances) or inside condition.

* The eyelids hang.

*The voice loses articulation.

*Positive outward appearances decrease;

*Awareness is more intense when the sound of the human scream is heard.

*Sensitivity to the social obligations of others diminishes.

You should remember that neuroception can either be related to the outside condition (e.g. an individual or situation that poses a risk to your life) or the inside condition. For example, fever, pain, or physical illness. Even low-level (rather that irate) facial influences can lead to neuroception of fear or threat and may even disrupt the advancement and unconstrained intuitive and complementary social commitment. An example of this is the level of discouragement experienced by a parent or the level of evil children. It can cause a loss of enthusiasm and a reduction in unconstrained, value-based social commitment.

Polyvagal theory: Three neural circuits regulate reactiveness

Is it possible to trace the roots of complex neurobehavioral patterns that enable people to have prosocial or cautious behavior? As we previously stated, all warm-blooded creatures, including humans must recognize an adversary and evaluate the security in nature. According to the polyvagal theory, vertebrates--particularly primates--have developed cerebrum structures that direct both social and guarded practices. Human conduct and physiology have been formed through the use of developmental powers. The evolution of the vertebrate nervous network has made it more complex and difficult. This phylogenetic progression has produced a nervous systems that allows people to communicate feelings, control and manage substantial and interpersonal states.

The theory of polyvagal interaction links the development a neural guideline of heart to full experience of feeling, passionate appearance, facial gestures, vocal correspondence and social conduct that is receptive. The theory suggests that the neural control system of the heart and the neural control systems of the facial muscles and the head are neuroanatomically linked.

The polyvagal theory shows three phases to the improvement of an animal's self-regulating nervous system. An unmistakable nervous circuit, which includes an autonomic nervous system, holds steady each one of the socially significant and flexible methods.

1. Immobilization

*Feigning passing, social shutdown.

*The most crude segment, which is imparted to most vertebrates.

*Depends in the most seasoned segment of the nerve vagus (an unmyelinated area that begins in a part of brainstem called the dorsal motor core of vagus).

2. Mobilization

*Fight-or-flight practices.

*Related to the function of the nervous system of thought, a system associated with increasing metabolic movement, and expanding cardiovascular yield (e.g. quicker pulse, greater heart rate contraction).

3. Social correspondence and social commitment

*Facial articulation, vocalization, tuning in.

*Dependent on the myelinated vis, which begins in the brainstem zone known as the coreambiguus. The myelinated nervous system suppresses the effect of the mindful nervous system on the heart and encourages quiet conduct.

For children as young as three months old, parents and grandparents need to set up social commitment systems to foster positive social connections. We at the University of Illinois at Chicago have developed a model which combines social responsibility to connection and the arrangement of Social Bonds through the accompanying advances.

1. Three neural circuits that are highly characterized support social commitment practices and mobilization.

2. Independently from cognizant mindfulness. The nervous system assesses nature's chance and determines versatile conduct. This coordinates the neuroception of a situation that may be sheltered, harmful, or life-threatening.

3. A neuroception is essential before social engagement practices can be made. These practices are enhanced by the benefits of the physiological state, which is related to social aid.

4. Social practice related to nursing, proliferation, and development of solid couple bonds requires immobilization unbefraid

5. Oxytocin - a neuropeptide that is involved in the formation of social links - makes immobilization conceivable by blocking protective freeze practices.

NEUROCEPTION/MENTALHEALTH DISORDERS

Neuroception that works is what we've been studying up until now. In a perfect scenario, a baby's understanding of her condition is enough to show that it protects her from being investigated. However, regardless of her neuroception warning her--precisely or otherwise--of potential danger from a "terrified, alarming" parent figure the baby can still take some preventative measures. What happens if neuroception becomes obstructed? One possible explanation for a few mental disorders is flawed neuroception. This is when the brain is unable to detect whether someone is reliable or nature is protected.

*The areas of the worldly brain that are accepted to stop fight, flight, freeze or flight are not activated by individuals with mental illness or schizophrenia.

*Tension disorders and despondency can lead to social dysfunction. The difficulties in controlling pulse and facial expression are evidenced in the vagal control of your heart and decreased facial expressiveness.

*Maltreated and systematized kids with responsive relational apathy will typically be either uninhibited (emotionally and physically inert) and/or restrained. These two conduct types are indicative of broken neuroception.

The research into children living in Romanian halfwayhouses has inspired enthusiasm for responsive relational issues, as well as the discovery of ways to remedy the disturbing influences on their social advancement. If these children's conduct suggests a defective neuroception in the earth, can there be any highlights that might allow them to feel more safe and push toward more common social conduct?

An investigation of Romanian babies being raised in a halfwayhouse shows how neuroception can be used to help improve connection practices. Analysts compared the two types of regulated children with those who were not systematized. One of the regulated children (the Standard Unit) was assessed according to winning norms. There were 20 different guardians working turning shifts, and around 3 parental figures per 30 children. The pilot unit consisted of ten children and four parent figures. If we apply neuroception to this examination, then we can conclude that children's ability to recognize guardians is essential to their neuroception of wellbeing. This, in turn, will be important for the advancement and proper conduct of society. It is important that children are able to discern the faces, voices, and developments of their guardians. This will help them to understand the importance of social commitment and the limbic system.

The Smyke et.al. Our speculation is supported by the information from the Smyke et. al. The greater the number of parents children had contact with, and the higher the rate for responsive relational difference among them, the more likely it is. The children in the standard unit were more likely than those from the other gatherings to have emotional issues that could be addressed. The responsive emotional issues of some children in the pilot-bunch were similar to those of children who hadn't been standardized. These discoveries suggest that understanding the relevant social highlights that limit the neural circuits, which intercede protective conduct system, can be used to "improve" prosocial behavior.

We at the University of Illinois at Chicago are using a newly grown organically constructed conduct intercession, based on standards obtained from the Polyvagal Theory. This method is being tested with children with mental disorders and those who have social correspondence or language difficulties. Our model assumes for certain children with social correspondence deficiencies (including those diagnosed to have chemical imbalance), the social commitment system is neuroanatomically as well as neurophysiologically unblemished. These children do not engage in intentional prosocial acts. Mediation must be used to activate the neural circuits of the brain that control the muscles and faces. The polyvagal theory predicts that when the cortical guideline and brainstem structures related to social commitment is enacted, social behavior and correspondence will rapidly happen as common new properties. Mediation "invigorates" or "works out", the neural pathways connected to tuning in. It also activates the functions of various parts of social commitment system. Acoustic stimulation is applied to the mediation. It has been modified PC to adjust the neural guidance of the middle ear muscles. Hypothetically it is suggested that the center ear muscles need to be managed during tuning. The nerves that control these muscles are connected the nerves of the face and heads that control social commitment. These are fundamental outcomes that are encouraging. They suggest intercessions designed to improve unconstrained socio conduct should: (1) guarantee a neuroception in members that will allow for the social security system to function; 2) practice the neural guideline to the social service system.

Chapter 5: Children, Emotional Resulation And Polyvagal Thory

As parents, we have a responsibility to help kids deal with all the situations they may face. This isn't an easy task. It is difficult to feel activated in kids' large feelings, even if they are outrage, dread, and pity. This is especially true for children who have trouble expressing these feelings. The polyvagal theory gives Parents the ability to look into your youngster's very enthusiastic states.

You may find your child resisting, refusing to be still, lying or being forceful towards parents or family. Parents are expected to work with their children to achieve desired outcomes. In any case, it can become a battle for wills. Parents would prefer not being the first to give. While it is important to set limits for our children and ourselves, it's essential that we help them loosen their passionate dysregulation in the safety of a mindful partnership.

Polyvagal Theory is an neurobiological system for understanding the link between brain, body and feelings. As we gain deeper understanding, our ability to sympathize with and effectively support children's passionate guides is increased.

A sentiments analyst

Adults can assist youngster with managing their passionate reactions to life. There will be times when you need to assume the role of investigator to discover the reason your child is in pain. Is it hunger or insufficient sleep, tactile based, a schedule adjustment, kin elements, or a school event?

Parents who have children who are dysregulated inwardly often feel upset. If your child is feeling stressed, you may feel worried for them and might even be questioned about your parenting skills. It's normal for young children to be angry at you or frightful towards you. These actions can cause feelings of hatred towards your child if they are repeated frequently. This doesn't mean that you should be disregarded by your child.

Polyvagal theory & kids

It is common for children to have difficulties communicating their emotions verbally. Some children can hold strong feelings in their hearts. Some of these children withdraw and stop socializing with others. Others may be more dangerous. These kids may become angry, causing them to have violent fits. In some cases, children can be violent towards relatives. Other family members may get hurt by their kids picking at their hair. Parents may find these behaviors disturbing. These practices are also used by children to control their body, mind, and emotions.

Researches have shown that the vagus neuron in the body controls elements of the autonomous sensory system. The brain interfaces with significant structures such as the stomach, gut, heart and lungs, throat and facial muscles via the vagus neuron. According to polyvagal theory there are three types of vagus neuron: one is responsible for thinking activities and one reacts for parasympathetic functions. The third, or social sensory system, controls and directs the activities. Let's take a look in greater detail at these parts.

The social sensory systems are related to connection, tranquility, well-being, and attention on what's happening right now. This vagus nerve is responsible for exhausting the face. It can be seen in children's eyes through a shimmer, grin and confidence in their ability to reach the rest of their world. Social connections are an important part of the social sensory network and help children explore their parasympathetic or thoughtful sensory systems.

It is linked to high excitement and preparation for developmental. If children are hyperactive, anxious, scared, squirmy and wiggly, then you can feel thoughtful actuation. This is known as a battle response or flight reaction when you feel dangerous or compromised. This can help prepare you for the play, if the social sensory system supports it.

The parasympathetic system is involved in low excitement levels, unwinding, withdrawal and sadness. The parasympathetic sensory system is responsible for children feeling weak and vulnerable. However, children can feel secure if they have their social sensory system upheld. Kids can be embraced by a pet or relax with calm fulfilling activities like reading or drawing.

Parents should be aware of the polyvagal theory in order to encourage the development and integration of social sensory systems in their children. This will help them to become more adjusted.

Spared with the ball

Here's an individual story to show how we can use our feelings to manage our children.

After a tough day, my request was that the children be allowed to use the lounge room. None of the children were listening. Instead they began to quarrel among themselves, contesting who created more chaos. We were all angry. I had used up all of my rationale. I felt the weight of my disappointment. I felt the drive to shout. I took a deep inhale, looked around and realized that the soccer balls made all the differences. Instead of venting my emotions on the children, i went to the ball and enthusiastically declared, "Soccerball, you're not going in the crate!" I'm so annoyed with your soccer ball. I don't hear you. The children and myself laughed at the ridiculousness of me shouting at the ball. I requested that they do it again. They started telling the different toys that their toys weren't going onto the racks. We began to work together in caring for the toys, and vigorously argued with the toys regarding why they wanted to go to sleep.

Tools to guide passionate people

It is my goal to help children realize that emotions are possible and can still be safe, loved, and alright. Here are some things that I suggest for children who are struggling with their behavior.

Do a self-check before you go: On a plane, there are guidelines that will help you to place your device on the first. Accept this guidance. Question: What way would you define yourself as being initiated? How would your language sound? How is your nonverbal communication communicating? What are your needs right now? You might have to stretch, inhale or call someone to help you feel connected and safer. To address the concern that your child is putting their safety or the safety of others, all options should be considered. But, it's important to recognize that your best defense is your kid. Self-guideline should be used as a test. However, practice is key in demonstrating your abilities to your child. For instance, you could say, "Whew!" I will take in a deep breath, then move my feet. That is so much more satisfying...

Be a feeling-criminologist. What is their nonverbal communication saying to you? What method is your kid currently using to manage feelings? How can you help your youngster experience connection? This will improve the social sensory system.

High excitement apparatuses. This is a great way to get your kid excited. For example, you might let them push against you and hold on to a pad. You could also use your rich swords for battle. I often tell my kids that outrage comes from a solid feeling. We need to find a good way to let it out. My child likes to strike a pad while he expresses his anger to me.

Low excitement: If your child pulls back or is close to you, make sure they allow you to come forward. You can use your voice tone and your breath to tell your child to give it a second thought. My little girl would like to get covered up if she becomes too powerful. My task in those minutes is just to calmly sit by her and inform her that I am there. She will end up on my lap, which is critical.

How to find skilled assistance

It's a sign to seek additional help when our relationships with our children are strained. If this happens, it's a sign to be more aware of your kid and their practices. This does not necessarily mean your child will experience withdrawal or sensory problems. In some cases, you may need to seek out more prominent symptoms for appropriate mediations. Information and aptitudes can only take us so far, especially when we are parents of children. Analyst and essayist, my goal is to dis-trash psychotherapy. It's often about lowering and agonizing at the thought of asking for help. Sometimes, it is possible to give people the greatest blessings: competent help for themselves and their children.

Are Children naturally resilient?

It is important to have faith in your children's ability for handling life's difficulties. We don't want them to feel overprotected. If we parents jump in too fast to deal with our children's problems, we can limit their ability for critical thinking. As they learn how to solve problems, children develop an ability to be creative and accept that they have an influence on their reality. The world in which we live isn't always kind and safe. It is difficult for our kids to manage this complex world.

Kids often need help when they are facing a challenging life situation. It is best to not overestimate a child's capacity to deal with stressors and other challenges. Not supporting children to cope with horrific accidents can lead to a loss of social, intellectual, and scholarly potential.

"In a perfect place, we give kids enough help and guidance to allow them to have fun and be challenged.

How to raise resilient kids

Flexibility can be defined as our ability adapt to any situation, even misfortune. As a quality-based psychotherapist, I would like to learn more about how flexibility can be used in my work with families. Caring Adults support children to become flexible and understand their world. They help them feel more competent in their passions, intellectual development, and social interactions.

We can help our children grow by being emotionally supportive parents. Adults who care and can help kids express their emotions effectively are the best support for them.

Younger children may have a better way to communicate with adults by drawing or playing.

Children older than 18 years old benefit from discussions that explore feelings and troublesome choices. They also learn how to examine the consequences kids make of their encounters.

A Curve Ball is thrown to you by Children at the moment.

Parents can feel scared and angry when they are around a child who is having a battle. Particularly when:

"My kid will not rest or stay awake!"

"My child hits his older sister or me with forceful words!"

"My little girl used the to be fine and dandy to go to class, and now she sticks and isn't discreet from me when it comes to first grade!"

"My youngster is blocking and simply won't listen!"

Every now and again, we have to respond or close off our children due to awkward feelings and feelings of trepidation. Pushing our children away or running from them is an instinctive and natural reaction to being anxious. To be fair, I welcome you see your kid's "curveballs" as a call to draw your child in, to look beneath the conduct and to associate with their inner world.

Realizing that you can experience outrage sometimes when you are defenseless or apprehensive can help your child to be more compassionate towards the troubling behaviors that arise from their vulnerability and fears.

Parents also need strength

For Parents, strength allows them to adapt imaginatively to the problems inherent in raising children. Parents need to have support. We can rely on the kindness of others, Parents, and advisors when necessary. These help us in investigating deeper topics and possible connections to the past. Being a strong Parent

Implies:

Get backing so your kids can win from your deterrents

Accepting your faults is part of learning to be more kind towards your kids.

Recognizing the fact that you don't know all the correct answers is key to allowing your kids to feel lost or confused.

Be aware that you want to be loved for your identity.

You will be told by pilots that the Adults should first use your breathing apparatus. If you are unable to do so, then help your youngster. The same is true for versatility. Adults who feel better are better able to assist their children.

Strength Informed Treatment

As individuals, we could all get "stuck" at times. There is no need to feel embarrassed or embarrassed about seeking help for your child. Flexibility educated therapy believes that children and parents should feel safe and secure so they can be able to contribute to their creativity, quality, and ability in dealing with life's challenges.

Chapter 6: Trauma, The Flaw Of The System

Trauma can effectively throw this whole system out of whack.

Remember how the vagus neuron affects several organs? This includes our heart, intestines and lung. The body also has a large influence from the parasympathetic nerve system. When we feel threatened, our sympathetic nervous systems kicks in and the parasympathetic is practically eliminated. That is where anxiety and other problems originate. Parasympathetic nervous is equipped with its own defense force in times when danger presents itself.

Our Biobehavioral defenses

Biobehavioral Defenses help us when we feel unsafe or threatened. In order to protect our safety, we will turn to these defenses if we aren't secure.

We will first use the sympathetic nerve system to bring us to self-protection. That means we will feel anxious, shaky, and panicked.

When the sympathetic nervous isn't working, we'll jump to the dorsalvagal complex. This is a primitive way to have defense strategies in place. This is where disassociation can occur, along with fainting and dizziness.

The vagus nerve, which is basically a brake, is essential for our body. We will become more susceptible to stress and experience a higher heartbeat if we remove it. The social nervous is the refined brake that helps to ease the effects of heart rate variability. This can lead to an increase in health and wellbeing.

The vagal brake is the dorsal vagal complex. The dorsal brake can lead to mental and physical disorders such as PTSD.

Trauma: How it works

A fight or flight can be triggered by traumatic past experiences. If this is a situation that you deal with daily or your environment exposes you to it, you will then experience a permanent fight or flight.

You may feel afraid doing chores like cleaning your house or raking leaves.

Trauma survivors often feel that their fear does not go away. They can't stop feeling like their bodies are on high alert.

You have to be anxious. Your vagal brake won't function if you have an elevated heart beat, respiration, or later, that can lead into heart disease, tachycardia, or both.

This can make it difficult to feel secure and unsure what to do. If you are suffering from trauma, it is likely that you won't be able to move past it. This could have serious implications for your physical well-being.

Social Nervous system Re-Engaging

Anxiety may be caused by your fight-or-fight mechanism being in control. You can't even concentrate on your own life. Your sympathetic nervous is in control, making you feel anxious and overwhelmed.

However, depression is also a result of this. While we will be discussing how the Polyvagal Theory may play a role in your depression, the real reason you might feel depressed is because your social systems haven't kicked into gear. You are just fiddling about, uncertain of what you should do, and unsure how to get there.

Most times though, your sympathetic nervous is activated when you're anxious. As the stress hormone cortisol builds, you'll feel the urge move when you're anxious. You can calm down by engaging your social nervous. Although it might seem counterintuitive, there are some ways that you can activate the social nervous system. We'll get to those later.

You may feel your parasympathetic nervous sistem mobilize when you feel down. If you don't know how to react to a trauma event and feel unsure, or you try to flee but can't, then you might be frozen.

If someone has trauma they can't get away from or anything they can do about it, they may feel frozen. That's because their parasympathetic nervous network is in place.

The problem is that this system will be activated only if you find yourself in an extremely dangerous situation. Problem with this system is, however, that you might not always realize that you're not actually in immediate danger.

We'll speak more about this in the section involving PTSD. Often, if both you and your situation aren't in control, and you're not engaging with your social nervous, you'll struggle to see the difference.

To overcome trauma you have to realize that the situation is not right now. You must nurture your relaxation response, and make that work. The problem is trauma. Until you can harness the emotion and not let it affect your life, you will feel it regardless of how you feel.

You may find it difficult to forget the past and difficult to harness your nervous system. This can have a significant impact on your life. A social nervous system malfunction can lead to dangerous heart conditions such as heart disease and even death. Understand that the body puts this there to help you fight danger.

These evolutionary systems were used back when we wanted to get away animals that might harm us. But the problem with evolution is that we've evolved. The reality is that trauma causes our bodies to respond on a stimulus/response basis. The best thing is that you can control it.

Can We Read Danger Cues?

Yes. Porges calls this neuroception. It is a process that the neural circuits read danger cues. As a result, we see the world around us in a way that allows us to judge whether it's safe or dangerous. This is often happening without us even knowing. This is a normal thing our bodies do. Natural scanning will help us.

Both sides of vagus nerves can be stimulated. But, from this, we are essentially scanning for information, and processing it with social interactions. This third component is stimulated. This basically means that we're mostly just scanning the information and checking it again.

The ventral part will focus on safety cues, such as physical safety and emotional security.

The dorsal part shows how we respond. It will tells you to get away. The last is, however, evidence that our dorsal vein system has taken over.

The Steps Trauma Must Take in the Nervous Network

Trauma is a complex process that can cause us to feel certain things. At the beginning, you may only see something that may stimulate your fight or flight system or cause us to shut down. Perhaps it's just something we see at first. As an example, suppose you are playing a game that requires us to feel scared and then we suddenly faint. People who are afraid of blood may actually be bypassing the fight/flight system. They don't feel the distress or fear, but instead they shut down and go to sleep.

Let's use another example. Let's imagine that you have to deliver an impressive speech. It's an extremely important component of your grade, so you're worried about how to deliver a compelling speech people love. Our body reacts to the moment we are on the stage. Instead of feeling scared we feel like we're going to faint. This is because your nervous systems bypasses socialization. Then, you take the easy way out and just...shut down.

Regardless of your reason, you will suddenly feel incredibly afraid.

The problem is that our body immediately identifies this as trauma. Our brains are conditioned to think, "That's a bad place. We need to get away!" It's impossible, so let's freeze up! That's how people freeze up in difficult situations.

Trauma does not have to be serious. Maybe you're afraid to speak to someone. This can cause you to freeze up, or even faint, and make it difficult to talk with someone. Our bodies will shift from thinking in a rational manner to shutting down. This could be a frightening situation. Perhaps there are good reasons to be scared.

No matter the cause of the event, our brains automatically go into fight, flee, or full shut down mode. It is so scary that the brain believes this response to be valid.

Our system's flaw is its inability to distinguish between real, threatening danger from danger coming from our brains. If you can recognize it, you will be able build a better mind and body, and learn to overcome traumas and fears that have been experienced all the way to this point.

You must learn to embrace your trauma and learn how to heal. The next chapter will address how to manage your social nervous and emotional traumas.

Chapter 7: Connecting With Your Higherself

Many people today wander blindly, searching haphazardly for their Higher Selves or meaning. They feel so disconnected from their lives, their people, and their callings that they are constantly changing their path without even thinking about it. Understanding why you feel fearful or depressed about the world is key to the current panic over stress disorders. This article will provide you with a framework that can help you align with your Higher Self, as well as an opportunity to acknowledge the relationship if you have it. This is the way you will drive your life forever if you are that connected. Your meaning in life is clear. Follow the path and your life will flow smoothly with grace, comfort, and joy. It is important to point out that not many people are able identify with the Self. The notion of personal clarification dominated society, while some blurred communities maintained some spiritual links. It should be consolation to you that you are one of the millions who suffer the same moral uncertainty, while courageously seeking out what few others have done, which is possible.

Your Higher Self Would Like You To Be Happy

Your Higher Self will need you to feel connected and comfortable. Your belief that pain and suffering on Earth is normal and necessary was incorrect. You were also expected make the most of contradictions in order to fill your days, weeks and months. Recognizing that it's normal to experience stress and problems and accepting the fact that there may be valid explanations. Your Higher Self can learn from all interactions. But it also acknowledges the habits and behaviors that you have at lower frequency levels. It is also aware of the lessons learned that will drive you toward these goals. It has all your secrets and talents. Even though you don't know it yet, you are still conscious of your infinite multidimensional existence.

Harmonizing with your Higher Self is Key

The secret to aligning your Higherself is simple, but not often mentioned. When you are in harmony with yourself, you can communicate your Higher Self. When you recognize this emotion, you can control the course of your emotions and strive to sustain it. Your thoughts can embed all of your positive and negative body emotions. Your body will feel strong when it's healthy. Your emotions will match your higher self's strength. Emotions that are weak or unbalanced would make your body feel "down" and cause you to feel inaccurate. The alignment key to your life is now. You know love, unity. Satisfaction, excitement, goodwill, goodwill, exuberance and joy. At that time you were fully identified with your higher self. People forget that harmony is possible when events happen in their favor. They're too busy to enjoy the joy of living, which is after all, the purpose of life. People often talk about coordination in the worst situations, but it is also most important.

Your heart can tell when you're in alignment

The process of aligning with your higher self is different for each person. However, the end result is always the same. You can feel it because your heart and body are free. You also have the option to feel like you are floating in air or lightening up. Your body can experience a sense of well being and attachment. It may also have the potential to spark development. With a gentle touch on your spine, unexpected joy or happiness can be achieved. There's no denying that there is truth to this. Connecting with your higher Self is the only way to be on top of everything. Your body is your representation of that. Everything feels in control, and you feel purposeful. It can be hard to resolve and overcome old and current political, family, and social structures. However, your body is the most valuable gift. Your body is the most powerful resource available to help you decide if you're compatible with your higher self.

Identifying Comforts/Discomforts

You need to know how your body reacts to pain. Most people feel better around the stomach and in other areas of the digestive track. These issues are usually caused by misalignment or alignment with the higher self. If you are out of balance, you may feel heavy, pressured, or have heartburn. Some people may experience discomfort in their lower back or shoulders. Several may get headaches. The best spiritual mentors are the strongest physical obstacles. When you experience pain, you can communicate with your higher self via a peaceful exercise. It may take you a while to truly understand what your Higherself is trying to teach through the body. It is important to take deep breaks and relax during painful moments so that you can develop and improve. Bravely ask your higher self for the information your body needs and be open to receiving it. You can feel, smell, taste, hear, see, and hear the reaction depending on your sensing tenderness. Your instincts are a powerful tool that can be unleashed courageously. You might get the response immediately, or even if it takes longer than you expected. It is essential to be aware that all questions are answered once you have been informed.

Wisdom of Your Body

Your Higher Self is your guide and teacher. He or she can provide you with great insights and guidance through your body's experience. Ask yourself questions while you meditate such as:

Am I afraid for the future

Is it in the best interest of me to work at this company?

Is my heart closed because I am afraid to have intimacy with my husband/work friends/other?

Is it in the best interest of me to pursue this relationship/course d'action?

Should I do something else with my life than I am doing now?

If you ask yourself any question, your body will answer it in one of these ways: 1) equilibrium (yes) and 2). It may warn you that something is not right (no more questions are required). You might then be able to recognize reality.

Complex Problems

Once you are able to tell the difference between yes and no questions, it is time for more difficult issues. While you are in quiet meditation, try to place your higher Self into a troubling situation. If you feel it's better to explain, write it down. Next, ask the question. If you ask the question, your body will answer with an emphatic Yes. You might want to tell your body NO or ask for more information if it's not aligned. Many people who are patient and flexible enough will ask and respond to these sessions, before going through an intense emotional and/or energetic release. Once you have learned a lesson, you can forget about emotional pain and unhappiness forever. This technique requires patience. People hate to learn their reality. The sensation is near the emotion until it gets forced into the stomach of a giant, knife-harpy unknown beast. Ask yourself why you fear the facts. The answer is likely to shock you. The unknown is necessary and important in spite of your doubts. All creativity comes from the unknown. Others wonder whether trusting the Higher Self with anything comes with risk. You don't always know where to go and you don't believe yourself. Many people have been taught that comfort is not something they can do. Your greater Self however, knows, regardless of circumstances, what must be accomplished in your mortal world. He or she will not take you to places that are impossible within your current life. Whatever someone says, as long as it feels good to your body, it's good. Get to know your Higher Self by looking into your own body. It's the most important investment you have ever made.

Sit Still

Find a quiet, quiet place to sit for a moment. Allow your purpose to be in contact with the Spiritual self, to offer yourself to it. You will gain its compassion, inspiration and all creation. Since the link to the Spiritual Self is beyond the subconscious mind, silence is a key element of this cycle. You must remove as many obstacles from your path as possible. Although you may not feel like you have made contact, it is important to not let this discourage you. It is your desire to communicate and receive direction, strength, and encouragement from your Divine Self that you must use this connection. It always addresses your questions.

Let Your Thoughts Fly

You can let go of all your thoughts, believe in eternal knowledge, unconditional Love and all-knowing Wisdom and open your eyes. Be still aware of the "I", pure consciousness. In a moment of inner silence, your mind will drift off to nothing. The Divine God will help you to let go of any negative feelings and bring you closer to Yourself. If you are able to let go of any thoughts or convictions that may hinder your ability to connect with your Divineself, it will make it easier to reach out to and accept your Divine Self.

Speak to the Divine Self

If you fall into silence ask for direction, wisdom or an answer. You have two options: you can speak softly or whisper it in your mind. In quiet moments, your Spiritual Self will show you the greater amount of wisdom and strength as well as devotion. These quiet moments can bring out new feelings of love and devotion for your Holy Self. This brings you more energy.

Be open

Inward greetings will then be sent that sound exactly like regular letters. Communication can come in many forms: energy, calmness, internal awareness, an answer to a question, deeper breathing, or through other means. It is perfectly fine if your answer is not clear or identifiable. You have received wisdom, extra strength, motivation, and the ability to unfold your destiny at just the right moment. This meditation is easy to do and you don't need to spend too much time. It can be used 10 to 22 times per day. Even taking a break after a busy day to ask for help or encouragement can be a great way of getting back to your Spiritual Selves.

Chapter 8: Functions Of Vagus Nerve

The vagus nerve controls the functions of all major organs. Let's not forget about the vagus nerve's unique functions.

Natural Inflammation Treatment

Vagus nerve stimulation can treat inflammation. It can also stop inflammation. It can also prevent inflammation from occurring. This is normal.

If your inflammation is excessive, you may be at risk for developing certain conditions. There are many conditions that can cause excessive inflammation such as celiac, autoimmune disorders, rheumatoid, and even sepsis. The vagus neuron has a network fibers that runs near your organs. Inflammation can cause the brain to release neurotransmitters called anti-inflammatory substances that will help regulate the immune system. The vagus nerve can be affected by overstimulating or not working correctly. This can increase the severity of inflammation and make certain conditions persist for longer. Fear and Vagus Nerve

Fear is something all of us experience at one time or another. If you've ever felt fearful in any situation, the vagus neuron is responsible. When you feel fearful, the vagus will transmit that information directly to your brain. Your brain will then receive the signal from the vagus and warn you. Your fight or flee response is activated.

You feel something in your stomach? The vagus neurom is probably at work. Your vagus will sense fear and report back any fearful feelings. Anxiety and other problems can arise from a overstimulated vagus neuron. Your response to life situations will be affected by the functioning and stimulation of your vagus nervous.

Vagus Nerve & Memory

Did you realize that the vagus nervous can also aid with memory? Research from the University of Virginia has shown that the stimulation of the vagus can lead to memory strengthening (Adelson & Associates, 2004). This is because the vagus nervous sends signals that the brain can detect a range of events and messages to it when it's stimulated correctly.

You release norepinephrine when you remember something. This neurotransmitter is deep in the amygdala where memories are stored. This could be why you feel a numb feeling in your stomach when you're fearful. The vagus neuro records your emotions and helps you recognize when it is time to get scared again.

Controls Relaxation

Vagus nerve is what triggers relaxation. Your vagus nervous system will tell your body to relax if it feels the fight or run response from the sympathetic nervous systems. Your vagus neuron is responsible to pump out acetylcholine. Acetylcholine is the hormone that tells you to relax. The vagus and sympathetic nervous systems pump out adrenaline or cortisol.

This nerve can tell many parts your body to relax when they're experiencing high levels stress. It's incredible! The vagus nerve can be thought of as a control point, which is responsible for all functions of the body. It communicates with different parts of your body when enzymes or proteins must be released. Vasopressin, used to reduce water loss, oxytocin for pain relief and prolactin for milk secretion, are just a few of the many chemicals your vagus nervous secretes. The vagus nerve is important because it controls many hormones.

Monitors Our Gag Reflex

The vagus nervous also stimulates your gag reaction. Your vagus will activate your gag reflex when something goes down the wrong pipes. You are likely to get a cough. The ear canal can be used to stimulate the cough reflex. The chances are that your cough reflex will trigger if something is in the ear canal. These reflexes protect your body from harm and keep it safe.

Sweat Control

The vagus neuron also controls sweat. Your vagus neuro will let you know when your body is too hot and make sweat to cool it off. You might also feel excessive sweating if you are anxious. Sweating can sometimes be a sign to leave the situation that you're in. The stimulation of the sweat glands within your body is controlled by the vagus neuro, which in turn controls your heartbeat and hormones.

Detecting the skin of the ears

The main vagus branch of this nerve is called the auricular. It is specifically involved with the detection of the skin of our auricles, tragus and the outer sound-related field of our ears. This branch's primary function is to sense sensation. We can feel temperature, pressure, temperature and dampness in the focal segment. Clinically, this branch is significant and applicable, since it is where the VN can easily be animated, such as with needle therapy.

Allowing food to be savored

If you're eating a feast, you might be thinking about the other thing. It's the way towards gulping each bite and stopping the breathing reflex with a goal to not choke. This important task is managed by the vagus neuron. The second portion of the VN (the vagus nerve) controls the functioning of five muscles in the Pharynx. This includes three constrictor muscles at rear of throat and two separate muscles that are associated with the throat.

These muscles are connected to the pharyngeal gulping period. This involves pushing bit nourishment towards the larynx or throat while keeping it away from the trachea. This VN section also covers the dynamic engine part the muffle response. This is a clinically important point, since poor vagus nervous capacity will result in hacking and an increase in the strength of the suppresser reflex. This reflex can be used for toning the VN via dynamic activities or locking in the muffle reaction.

Treatment of your Airway and Vocal Chords

Are you aware of the effort required to keep your upper-airway open each time you take a deep breath? You also need to use your vocal cords for this purpose. In the event that you have ever thought about what nerve is capable of ensuring that verbal correspondence with others around you is possible, it is the vagus. The VN's third- and fourth parts are the repetitive and prevalent laryngeal. For the muscles beneath the vocal string, the predominant laryngeal nerve is answerable while the repetitive one is for the muscles. The laryngeal superior branch is responsible for engine data, while certain muscles of larynx are not affected. It also controls pitch. The predominant laryngeal branches have a limited capacity which can lead to a pitch adjustment. Poor vagal tone in this region of the nerve can indicate a rough voice or a repetitive, exhausted voice. The nerve can also become irritated and dangerous, allowing food or drink to enter the trachea by the impairment of the vocal lines.

The repetitive branch of the larynx transmits engine information to the muscles below the vocal ropes. It allows sounds to shape by opening and closing the vocal rope structures. It also includes a tangible segment that transfers data between the throat, trachea and inner mucous layers. The breakdown of these nerves causes dryness, loss, and inconvenience when breathing is performed. These laryngeal muscle are responsible for the opening, shutting and capacity of the air route. Vagus nerve tone and diminished capacity would be responsible for breathing difficulties. The vagal capacity of your aircraft route is particularly affected by how you breathe and what tone your muscles are. Incessant obstructions to a good, efficient, and well-worked aviation route will result in a decrease in the capacity of these muscles. This will adversely influence your vagus nervous system's capacity.

Controlling Your Breathing

What about relaxation? All things considered the vagus also has a role in this crucial task. The VN's aspiratory function connects to and interfaces the thoughtful sensory system.

innervates trachea, bronchi and spleen of the two lung. The vagus section is a tactile neuron that transfers data from the brain to determine lung extension levels. This includes oxygen and carbon dioxide levels. The vagus nerve initiate eases breathing and extends breath. The rest-and ingest stage will have deeper breathing and come from the stomach, rather than extra muscles. The pace of breathing will also be lower. An individual will transition from a state of fight-or-flight to one that is rest-and-summary. A full, moderately fast breath rate will activate and stimulate the vagus neuron. Vagus tone, which is necessary for opening the aviation pathway in the pharynx or larynx and trachea, is vital.

VN's engine segments innervate muscle cells in the larynx and pharynx. Incessant obstructive pseudonymonic disorder (COPD), or obstructive napnea, can both cause an obstruction to the flight path. Both of these conditions signify low vagal tone. They also require vagus nervous enactment. I will even venture to such an extreme as to state that check of the aviation routes can be a potential main driver of vagus nerve brokenness--something that will be talked about in a lot more prominent detail in later parts.

Controlling the Heart Rate

Your heart thumps in order to receive oxygen-filled blood and replenish your cells with nutrients. Also, it can send poisons out to the organs that can eliminate them. The VN does a great job of keeping the pulse within a safe range, even when the body is under pressure. Without the VN, hearts would not function at their optimal rate. The vagus is easily associated with both the sinoatrial and the vagus hubs, which provide electrical signals to the two arries (the narrower chambers at high points in the heart). It is also linked to the atrioventricular, which manages siphoning and with the withdrawal weight of both ventricles (the two thicker councils at the bottom of the heart). The sympathetic nervous network activates the heart in times of fight or flight by increasing siphoning and compression rates.

Once the stressor has passed away, the body enters the rest-and–overview stage and moves towards a vagal implementation stage. The VN has parasympathetic fibers that regulate the pulse, and they also decrease siphoning compressions weight. These filaments are responsible for reducing heart activity. This allows the heart relax and recovers from stressors.

Maintaining an Optimal Blood pressure

The amount of liquid present in the circulatory tract is determined by pulse. The kidneys can filter liquid and poisons through the body. The vagus neuro transfers data to and fro the kidneys. This assists it in managing water and liquid progression inside the renal glomeruli. When the body's pressure is high, signals from the blood vessels (explicitly the carotid) are sent up to the brainstem for withdrawal to the renals via the vagus and thoughtful nervouss.

At that time, the kidneys contract their vessels and increase circulatory strain by decreasing the amount of water being passed through the circulation system. The carotid body signals the kidneys to increase circulation and sift through more fluid. These hormones work with the vagus as well as thoughtful nerves. The hormones work by controlling the nerves quickly and providing a steady, moderate administration.

Hypertension can be a sign of a serious condition. Meds are often prescribed to help control it. Hypertension can indicate an overactivation or stress hormones by the adrenal organs. It is also known as the stress reaction. The thoughtful nerves intercede through hypertension. It is also an indication of vagus nerve irritation and low vagal tone.

Controlling the Liver's Multiple Functions

The vagus nerve is responsible for transferring significant data from and to the liver. It also handles about 500 other errands. The most important capabilities of this area are not covered here. The liver controls the flow of bloodstreams through the body. During times when pressure is high, bloodstreams are pushed towards the arms and legs by the liver to expand muscle enactment. The liver will lose bloodstream, because assimilation of blood filtration is not necessary during such stressful occasions. When the body has reached rest and digest stage, vagus neuro enactment is increased in monitoring glucose levels through its pancreas. This serves as a trigger for the production, as well, the discharge of insulin. As blood glucose rises, insulin is generated and released from the pancreatic islet cells.

As glucose expands, insulin discharge increments. A spike of glucose will simply lead to an increase insulin's arrival. And, there will be no insulin opposition if the insulin levels continue to rise. Long-term diabetes will result, as previously described. A hormone called cholesterol (CCK), is released in the gut immediately after a meal. This triggers a vagus neuro, which signals the islet tissues to release insulin as necessary. To ensure that proper motion is achieved from the gut into the cerebrum as well as from the brain to to the pancreas requires vagus work. Inability to maintain a healthy level of functioning will eventually result in a state of sickness. We should be allowed to start the parasympathetic framework with consistency to prevent insulin obstruction and, eventually, glucose dysregulation and diabetes.

Problems with Digestive Enzymes Release from the Pancreas

The pancreas doesn't just manage glucose; it also delivers and discharges stomach-related compounds to the small digestive system, in light of a feast.

Our small digestive system and our taste buds send signals to our brains when we eat. This helps us determine the specific macronutrients in the meal. Is the feast high in protein, fat, and possibly sugar? What proportion of each ha made it to the stomach? And how quickly did it make it there? Once the answers to these inquiries are resolved, the vagus flags the pancreas to discharge explicit stomach related chemicals--proteases, lipases, and amylases--to help in the breakdown of these macronutrients, permitting for processing and in the end the correct utilization of these supplements by our cells. If there is a greater amount of protein in the blood, the pancreas secretes proteases to break down the bonds among the amino acids. Because of higher levels of fat, the pancreas secretes Lipases to help break down triglycerides.

Amylase is released due to higher starch levels. It helps break down complex sugars, and converts them into basic sugars. Without this procedure, the body wouldn't be able to ingest significant macronutrients essential for cell growth. Amino acids play a major role in the creation of new proteins in our cells. They also act as receptors, synapses and receptors for certain intracellular flagging particles.

The unsaturated fats and simple sugars are used principally in vitality generation. Meanwhile, the cholesterol section of fats serves as the precursor for steroidhormones, such as estrogen, testosterone, and cortisol. This is because these particles are critical to cell function. Therefore, a perfectly functioning pancreas must ensure that these atoms can be absorbed into the body.

Overseeing Gut Motor Function

The vagus performs a vital job by moving food from the mouth into the stomach. After having taken a few bites of nourishment, the vagus then moves the food through the stomach. The vagus neuro pushes it to the next place when that nourishment, or the bolus, hits the rear part of the mouth. It is essential that the stomach-related muscles and sensors are functioning properly for this to happen. Each bite brings the mouth to the back of your throat. This triggers a stretch reflex, which sends signals to the brainstem using the vagus nervous. In turn, the VN signals to the smooth muscles cells for them to take part and push the bolus down. This process is known as peristalsis.

This seemingly simple capability is actually very complicated and essential because the stomach connected tract is so long. We need to develop along the stomach linked tract in order to extract nourishment from our nutrition and push out undesirable guests. A poorly conditioned VN could lead to blocked development of bolus in the tract. Inadequate vagal tone and the absence of essential enactment are both signs of poor bowel function. The most serious problems are when we don't eat well and eat too fast. This is the drive-through issue. It's when we eat quickly and in a hurry while being under intense pressure. We are attempting to initiate a rest-and-condensation process while in a fight-or-flight state. It is important to realize that nourishment can't travel this way from the pharynx, through the throat, into the stomach, and against gravity when the climbing or transverse colons are being moved.

Chapter 9: Clinical Utilizations Of The Polyvagal Hypothesis

The polyvagal hypotheses, which shows both the phylogenetically supported progressive system for autonomic states and specific triggers that can cause disintegration of this chain, provides another method for investigating unusual conduct. The hypothesis highlights that the mammalian sensorial system is not sensitive to natural requests or dangers. However, the hypothesis also suggests that the mammalian system will be able to quickly alter to neural mediated state upon an anticipated request. Different from models of psychopharmacology which also emphasize the importance and management of state, polyvagal theory highlights the neural systems that control the state and the request to which these neural components were inspired. The polyvagal hypothesis highlights the adaptability that the sensory systems can bring to the balance of the autonomic states. This view seems to be different regarding pharmacological techniques that are capable of changing the autonomic system without drawing in sensory systems. Another worldview based on polyvagal hypotheses has been tested. This worldview accepts that state can be modified in an expected way. These changes in the state would be related either to constraining or potentiating explicit practices. This new worldview recognizes that state changes are caused by shifts in neuronal guideline of autonomic apprehensive framework. However, explicit reactions are evoked by quantifiable enhancements.

One can see the world from a Z perspective. Manipulation; assessment of the autonomic system; and Z2 assessment and control of learning and social conduct. This worldview should enable one to predict that the scope, including PhysZ, of discernible practice will change as the environment for security driving the neuronal guideline of the autonomous sensory system (autonomic) is controlled. This worldview allows us assess the effects of explicit settings on an autonomic state's neural guidanceline.

While certain settings may promote solitary conduct (e.g., animosity and wellbeing Z. powerlessness), others might help with positive social conduct or wellbeing. This is because the sensory system's highlights can only be understood when the environment of the living person's connection with the condition is being used. An individual could be interfacing in an area that is not only inefficient in animating social behaviour and scholarly advancement, but also may be damaging to both metals and physical wellbeing. The polyvagal hypothesis limits us to view bargained socio-economic conduct from an alternative point of view. The hypothesis suggests that the physiological condition limits the scope of social conduct. The hypothesis emphasizes the possibility that assembly and immobilization techniques could be flexible systems for a terrified person. Z. It could be that creating conditions of calm and practising neural guideline brainstem structures can potentiate positive social behaviour by invigorating practice of the social responsibility framework. This third worldview or mediation worldview is based around organically-based practices. Z. Therapy and subjective therapies mediation methodologies. Acoustic incitement is used to improve social conduct. This method was then tested on children with mental disorders. The mediation was based on some standards that were determined from the polyvagal hypotheses. The first is the territory of ambiguous brainstem that controls Z, as well as Z through the militated Vagus. The head muscles, including the facial, centre ear, mouth and larynx. These muscles control facial signalling, looking, tuning into, vocalizing, and vocalizing. If this neural guideline is not valid, the facial features won't function. The face might need Z for facial expressiveness, eyelid open, prosody, and even listening. These facial highlights have been used to portray a few psychopathologies. Mental imbalance, discouragement forceful scatters, posttraumatic stress problem, enthusiastic states. During the serious exam, there will be pain, rage. outrage. sorrow. The central ear muscles do a significant job of separating the human vocal cords from complex acoustic conditions. The neural tone of the central ear muscles becomes low and the centre hearing structures don't have the ability to filter out low-frequency sounds. These low-frequency sounds are what command our advanced modern world's acoustic conditions. Even people with ordinary hearing can experience trouble tuning in, due to problems in their ability to hear the human voice.

Third, third, the neural line of the centre ears muscles is connected with the lines of different muscles on the face which control the outward appearance of vocal inflection. Incitement for improving neural guideline should coordinate with the other muscles of the face, which control facial expression, facial expression and vocalization. The brainstem nears the lower half of the cerebrum, which contains the lower engine neurons for the social commitment framework. It is important to note that social correspondence can be a bit more fitting than normal times. The upper engine neuron in the frontal cortical cortex directs the lower engines neurons when there is a need for appropriate social correspondence (e.g., facial expression, vocal pitch). The hypothesis suggests that these lower engine neural guides are displaced by phylogenetically less complex frameworks.

The cruder frameworks are susceptible to subcortical systems that advanced to arrange endurance. These structures oversee metabolic assets to advance assembly. Assets can be frozen or destroyed by immobilizing. The identity determines whether an individual can speak with the community or take part in a system that fights or freezes.

EFFECTS OF TRAUMA & ITS RESPONSES

In the case of an injury that is not certain, it may be possible to live with a constant battle or flight. It is possible to channel the battle or-flight tension through exercises such as cleaning the house or raking the forgottens. But these exercises will have a different vibe than they would if you had finished social commitment science. (Think "Whistle While You Work")

Some injured victims feel that their fight/flight instincts are not channeled by any movement. In the end, they feel trapped, and their body shuts down. These customers could live in a perpetual shutdown.

Diminish Levine was a long-lasting friend and associate to Porges. He studied the shutdown reaction through creature perceptions and bodywork. Waking the Tiger. Healing Trauma. He explains how to wake up from a shutdown. We can rise up in dangerous situations when we have shut down, and an opening for dynamic endurance appears. As advocates, we might perceive the shift from shutdown and battle to trip in a customer's movement from the gloomy into nervousness.

In any event, how can we assist customers in achieving their social engagement science? If our customers seem to be living in a constantly dissociative, discouraged, or shutdown environment, we can assist them with their transition into battle/flight. When customers feel the need to fight or fly, we should help them find a feeling that they are well. They will be able to move into their social obligation framework once they feel protected.

Customers can get out of shutdown and dissociative reactions using body-mindfulness therapies. These systems are both part of argumentative conduct treatment or intellectual conduct therapy (DBT). Customers can stop experiencing a shutdown reaction when they become more present in themselves and are more able to handle strong strain. CBT/DBT also includes idea rebuilding methods to help customers evaluate their own wellbeing and break down barriers. Intelligent listening methods are able to help customers establish a relationship with their advisors. This allows customers to feel enough safe to explore social commitment science.

The polyvagal hypothesis offers a possible stage to unravel social behavior inside a neurophysiological framework. The emphasis placed on phylogeny makes it possible to understand the progressive sequence of versatile reactions. The social commitment framework is more than just a way to make social contact. It also tweaks your physiological state in order to improve social conduct. The polyvagal hypothesis posits that social behavior is a new property of phylogenetic advancements in the autonomic sensory systems. Reliable with this progressive theory saw neural disintegration of the social correspondence and positive social conduct frameworks to the cruder fight. Flight and shirking. The hypothesis is not just useful for clarifying the pathophysiological causes of clinical disarrangements. However, it also helps to present a worldview that might have general applications to people with trouble in social behavior.

THE VAGAL AACTIVITY REGULATION, AND INTEROCEPTION

Your ability to accurately integrate and respond with interoceptive info is crucial for self-regulation. Interoception helps us to regulate our emotions, pain, addiction, and other adaptive behaviors that include social interaction. Interoception is essential for resilience because the correct processing homeostasis encourages a quick return to internal body balance.

Interoception is essential for:

The bridging of top-down, bottom-up processing.

In the evaluation and assessment of emotions, feelings, and sympathovagal balance. In the integration of cingulate, insular and solitary cortices:

Emotional input

Interoceptive input

Maintaining a good balance in sympathovagal function facilitates a more coordinated response from the person to mind and body as well as environmental phenomena.

The brain and the viscera have a constant conversation. The gut-brain relationship is a key facilitator in this conversation. It consists:

Top-down neural pathways

These pathways enable the central nerve system to control digestive functions within the gastrointestinal track. The luminal skin of the gastrointestinal track is 100 times larger in humans than the skin. Therefore, its complexity and extent are greater than skin and other organs.

This study has drawn a lot of attention in neuroscience, psychology and physiology to the effects of gastrointestinal processes on higher brain centre executive functions, motivated behaviour and affective states.

In addition to digestive and ingestive functions, gastrointestinal sensory information to the brain creates a neural basis of gut feelings. These feelings are what shape subconscious emotional responses to daily threats and opportunities. These threats and opportunities can come from either within the body or the environment. They produce complex circuits that organize the central nervous sistem's psychological, behavioural, emotional, and affective responses.

These responses could be from birth or can also be conditioned by learnings. They may also be subject to autonomic as well as endocrine modifications that can alter their visceral functions. It mainly involves GI functions, and interoceptive input to the brain. The interoceptive feedback from the brain about GI functions and other visceral elements strongly influences the cognitive-emotional processes that form motivated behaviour.

Bottom-up methods

These pathways enable the central nerve system to receive instant feedback about interoceptive visceral condition.

Interoceptive Feedback plays an important role in motivating behavior.

The vital homeostatic functions of the hindbrain spinal visceral Circuits and their interconnections. In which avoidance behaviour and goal directed approach arise from emerging cognitive and physiological challenges as well as anticipated outcomes.

Although there are many choices and decisions that can be made at any given moment, subconscious influences on motivated behaviours exist in the body. There are many fibres of the vagus nervous that monitor pre-absorptive and postsorptive points in the GIT.

Vagal control also correlates to differential activation at brain regions that regulate responses to emotion regulation.

Comparatively, low vagal regulation that is associated with maladaptive, top-down, or bottom-up processing leads to less behavioural flexibility.

Regulating vagal activity

Complex Ventral Vagal Complex

The social communication network, also known under the name ventral vagal system. It is the branch belonging to the vagus neural, which has soothing or calming effects. It facilitates social engagement. Ventral vagal complex creates a sense of safety in the environment.

A neural platform to support prosocial behavior

The neural regulation that regulates organ states can be used to influence social behaviour

Maintaining homeostasis while restoring fascial expressions

Both the expressive domains and the receptive realms of communication are included.

The motor component to vagal activity regulation arises in the nucleusambiguous. These regulate the muscles of your head, face and heart with the bronchi and the heart. These connections are a way for individuals to connect with others and encourage human engagement.

Ventral vagal pathways regulate vagal activity in areas where there is high cardiac tone. More, it involves adaptive bottom–up and top–down processes such as flexibility or affective processing of physiological system to respond to and adapt the environment.

Sympathetic Nervous System

It is associated with fight/flight behaviors which are primary or initial level defence strategies. In order to support mobilization behaviour, the body requires a high metabolic output. You will notice significant physiological changes in the recruitment of sympathetic neural system circuits. There is an increase and decrease in heart rate and respiratory rate, shunting and blood from the periphery, dilation and dilation, increased muscle tone, and inhibitions of gastrointestinal function.

The individual's ability to use their physiological resources to react to perceived or real dangers in the surrounding environment, and work towards safety and security is possible through the mobilization of these resources. This system can be associated with emotions such as fear and anger, which are used to manage the danger or protect.

Complexes Dorsal Vagal

It supplies the primary vagal motor fibers for organs beneath the diaphragm. This structure is considered the most primitive and is designed to withstand extreme danger and terror. It activates a passive response that results in a dramatic drop in cardiac output and reduced muscle tone.

The reduction of the metabolic demand for survival by inhibiting viscera is called immobilization. It can be described as either immobilization or shutdown. It can be associated with:

The freeze or collapse response.

Behavioural shutdown.

A feigning death.

The disembodied dissociative condition may include the loss or immobilization of consciousness.

In response to safety or threat, the neural platforms create a physiological situation that limits or allows the person to exhibit certain behaviours and emotions. Other attributes of ventral vagal complexity allow blended states with sympathetic nervous systems. The ventral valve complex can still be reached and functionally supports the subordinate systems. Ventral vagal complex becomes less functional and allows for the easy access to the sympathetic nervous as a defense mechanism. SNS can also block functional access to DVC shutdown. The shutdown reaction can lead to death if the SNS is not in control reflexively.

Vagal Afferents

Tone is important.

Provide steady streams of glutamatergic infusions to postsynaptic neuron cNTS.

Smooth muscle tone can be used to help you feel more alert.

Few peripheral axons from vagal afferents ramify inside the mesentery as well as in intramuscular arrangements in whole smooth muscular layers of the esophagus. Some vagal sensory Axons terminate at the interstitial Cajal cells, smooth muscle layer, and the Meissner/myenteric plexus in the enteric neuro system.

The 80% of the vagus neuron's afferent fibers are responsible for transmitting information about the environment and conditions to the brain. It is important that you note this, even though some vagal afferents have been classified as chemo/mechanoreceptor. Many of these are multimodal. These are capable of responding to a variety mechanical and chemical stimuli.

The variety of receptors that the vagal sensory nerves express is quite diverse. These are specialists in the detection, production, and monitoring of circulating and local gut hormones.

This way, the plasticity within the vagal neuron fine-tunes the major neural routes through which information about internal environment and ingested foods reaches the central nervous to influence behaviour.

The cNTS neural receives direct synaptic input and relayed information from the vagal-GI tract. All other sensory neurons can survive the visceral. This nerve is a crucial component of the parasympathetic nerve system. This nerve is a component of the autonomic neuro system.

The more robust the vagus responses, the more the human body can regulate blood sugar levels. This will reduce the likelihood of developing diabetes, cardiovascular disease, or stroke.

Low vagal tone has been linked to chronic inflammation. The process of neuroception, which isn't under voluntary control, has an effect on vagal nerve regulation.

Vagally Mediated Influences and Motivated Habits

Critically, survival of an individual depends on his ability and willingness to avoid potentially life-threatening situations. Motivated behaviours refer to the adoptive behavioural strategies that support these vital capabilities. Because they are motivational and can be activated, energized and directed towards a goal. It is closely associated with the emotional state of hedonic or euphoric states. They are broadly divided into two groups: approach and avoidance.

Motivated avoidance and approaches are motivated by learned associations as well as hereditary factors. Intrinsic variables include the rewarding characteristics of sweet taste and absorption, as well as the aversive nature of pain, nausea, and hunger. The learned associations refer to drug self administration, cuepotentiated nutrition, or the conditioned avoidance flavours that can be paired with gastric cancer. The complex circuits within the central nervous system that regulate the initiation of, processing and termination of motivated behaviors, guiding human beings, are remarkable conserved.

Attention to situations that maintain the internal climate

Keep away from anything that might pose a threat for your homeostatic requirements.

These highly evolved neural systems include key circuit Nodes at each level of the neuraxis. Every NODE receives interoceptive feedback signal directly or indirect from the CNTS.

Chapter 10: Parasympathetic System

The parasympathetic system is part of the autonomic neuro system (ANS). The parasympathetic system is not a true system. It is only part of the ANS. The history of the study into the anatomy of the ANS and physiology are full of reasons to classify the parasympathetic part of ANS as the ANS.

Now we'll be looking at the anatomy. We'll first look at cranial flow and then at the sacral output.

So it reduces contractility, the rate of heartbeat and causes bronchoconstriction in the lungs.

You can find the edinger Westphal nerve in the midbrain. The oculomotor nervous extends into the ganglion located in its periphery. From there, it creates the ciliary muscles and makes the pupil smaller. Next you have the salivatory nuclear nuclei. Here the superior salivatory branch of facial nerve is located inside the pons. While the inferior salivatory branch is in lower medulla. This nucleus provides postganglionic projections for the parotid.

The vagus neural is different. It does not have a peripheral motor nucleus in its head. Therefore, it originates at the dorsalmotor nucleus (vagus) in the medulla.

The heart beats 60 times per minute when you are at rest. However, it would be quite easy to change things if you disconnected your heart from your neuronal system. But your heart would not stop. It would be quite the opposite. It would accelerate.

It would beat around 100 beats/minute when it was still at rest. Your heart would beat at a rate two-thirds faster that normal before you even started to sweat. This would put a lot of strain on your cardiac muscle. The surrounding blood vessels would experience immense pressure. Your body would suddenly be under immense pressure and require, and waste, a lot o energy. This would basically mean that you would be out balance.

There are 12 of these brain nerves. Their contents vary depending on the type of neuron they contain. You're not only referring the autonomic systems, but also other motor fibers. Motor fibers can also be found in certain cranial nervous systems. They control voluntary functions like moving your eyeballs. Others have only sensory fibers and relay data to your sensory cells. For fun, some of the motor and sensory neurons in your cranial nerves are mixed. So which ones are there? And what do these 12 nerves do? As anatomists we need to know the wiring-diagram of the cranial nerves. We don't want our patients to feel like they are part of an action movie. SHOULD I KUT THE REDWIRE OR THE BLACKWIRE? It's probably not a good idea to cut any wires if you're inside someone's brain stem. To keep track of all 12 of these important cranial nerves, you'll need to use mnemonics. You will need to know the name of each one, including whether it's a motor or sensory nerve.

The map of cranial nerves is based on a ventral look of brain. That is, looking at its bottom, with the anterior on the top and the posterior on the bottom. Let's get to the names. To begin at the top, you'll encounter the olfactory, which is responsible for capturing scent information and sending it to your brain. This is followed by the optic, which receives visual data. Next, there is the oculomotor which controls four out of six muscles controlling the movements of your eyes.

The next nerve is located in the brain's middle ventral side. It controls one muscle of the eye. The trigeminal, the largest cranial neuron, is just below. It splits into three main strands (hence the 'tri'), and innervates your jaw muscles and facial skin. The abducens then stimulates the muscles in your eyes. It is followed by facial nerve which controls most facial expressions. Next, the auditory neuron. You probably know what this is for. However, you may be surprised to learn that the auditory and cranial nervous systems control organs at the front of your skull. This includes the eyes, facial muscles, and the mouth. As you move further down, however, the nerves begin to innervate lower and more posterior parts of the skull.

The glossopharyngeal nerve is what connects to your tongue, pharynx and mouth. Your vagus and pharynx nerves follow. The hypoglossal allows you to talk and swallow. It also lets you use your tongue and mouth for other functions. You have a lot to learn and many new words. How will you remember it all? Find a way to recall the first letter of each person's name in order. O-O-O ...? It doesn't really mean anything. One mnemonic you might hear in school is: On Olympus' tallest peak, a Fin viewed hops. This sounds quite strange and not very easy to remember.

Olympus I refer to? Fin? Hops? We science lovers of the 21st Century need something more. Perhaps Lord of the Rings-lovers might like to hear: Onward, Old Orcs! Go to the Argonath for a Great Villain Slay Hobbits! I'm just trying my best to help. Whatever tool you use for remembering the names of the various cranial nervous systems, you have to also track their functions. This is how you know if they are sensory, motor, or both. To remember, teachers often use this same sequence of S, M, and B. My brother claims that bigger brains matter more than my sister. This one isn't so bad.

I don't know, maybe it will be better for you to try something like this: Sorry! Sherlock -- Mean Moriarty beats Me, but Some Bobbies busted Master Moriarty masterfully You are free to develop your own. Please feel free to comment on them. This long nerve stretches from the brainstem all to the most important visceral parts of your body, including your heart and lungs. Vagus nerves operate as a two way street. They carry incoming sensory information through the peripheral system to brain and send outgoing motor instruction to the rest. It is called a B nerve because it has both motor function and sensory functions. Its functions are almost all automatic so you rarely notice it working. Imagine you've just experienced a very stressful day. Now your sympathetic system is energized. You arrive home, collapse on the couch and munch half a piece of pizza. Your stomach sends signals from your brain to the sensory nerve. Axons are located in your vagus neuro. They tell you that your stomach is full of protein, starch and fat. Your brain recognizes that your stomach has been churning, which can be a parasympathetic behavior, so it sends signals to your brain via the vagus neuro, triggering parasympathetic actions such as slowing your heart beat, putting some glucose into storage, and decreasing all of the norepinephrine released by your sympathetic system throughout the day. Soon, you'll feel more relaxed. That's just one reason eating can help you feel more relaxed. It can feel so good, that you might eat even if your stomach is empty.

As I have said before, it is easy to view the two divisions in your autonomic system differently or even as rivals. Your body should be viewed as a whole. You can see the two halves of a scale. It may look balanced in one corner, but it could also appear as if it were balanced on one side. This balance is what you call homeostasis. Sex is an important aspect of human life.

It falls within the parasympathetic area of "necessary and not an emergency." The parasympathetic is responsible for making sure you're calm enough that you can even consider having sex. They also have to funnel extra blood from your muscles to your pelvis, which can cause problems with sexual function. To keep you excited, you will also need a boost of the sympathetic nervous system. Both sides of the spectrum are important. The balance depends on how much of each you have. Your "sympathetic sound" and "parasympathetic sound" determine how fast action potentials are moving through each division. Most of the time, the parasympathetic sound is dominant, keeping down your sympathetic response. You need your parasympathetic to keep you heart rate steady and not racing like a rabbit's. It's also why most of us can do the eating, drinking, and sex-having that we enjoy.

Chapter 11: Borderline Personality Disorder And Emotion Regulation

Many individuals with marginal character problems (BPD) feel extraordinary feelings. The Diagnostic and Statistical Manual of Mental Illnesses 5th Edition (DSM-5), a booklet that provides human services, identifies many of the BPD side effects with feelings guideline issues.

What is Emotion Regulation?

Feeling guideline refers to a variety of ways in which an individual can identify with others and follow-up on those passionate encounters. This includes:

Your ability understand and accept their excited encounters

Your ability to use solid methods to control awkward feelings.

Your ability and willingness to accept appropriate practices in times of upset

Individuals with great feeling guidance abilities can control the desire to engage in incautious activities, such self-hurts, foolish conduct, physical hostility, and other behaviors under passionate pressure.

Case of Emotion Regulation against Deregulation

For example, someone who doesn't have BPD may experience a separation. She will likely feel hurt and perhaps discouraged but will still be able to control her feelings and continue her daily practice. She will attend class, but she will also get down to business.

BPD sufferers do not have the ability to properly manage their emotions. When he's in similar circumstances, he can become discouraged and stop working.

BPD and Emotional Problems

BPD diagnosis criteria include a majority of issues involving feelings. A portion of these include:

Rapidly changing mood swings, and irritability. People who have marginal character issues may have difficulties controlling their emotions and communicating their feelings. Emotional episodes are also quite rare. These episodes can cause problems with everyday activities such as pursuing a vocation or simply thinking about yourself. Other people may have trouble being around you during these scenes due to various reasons. It can also hurt your connections.

BPD sufferers frequently feel the void. They will try various activities to fill that void. No matter how many close friends or family they have, they feel isolated and miserable. BPD can be a vicious circle. People who have difficulty directing their feelings may lose friends. A feeling of forlornness can lead to a decrease in the ability to manage feelings.

Trouble Controlling Anger BPD can sometimes be triggered by small irritations or insults that can cause rage, leading to dangerous or brutal behaviors.

Suspicion & Fear of Abandonment - Individuals with BPD fear being dismissed or distant from others, leading to extreme neurosis. It can make them act out, and they may look for consolation. Unfortunately, some of the actions that are triggered by a need for consolation can drive people with BPD away.

BPD may cause difficulty in controlling feelings. This could lead to outrage or dismissal. Troublesome behavior can result from your inability to control your emotions. This can have a negative impact on your relationships and ability to integrate with your loved one.

How to Deal With Your Emotions when You Have BPD

BPD is a condition that can make feeling like a guideline difficult. However, it is easy to master this aptitude and get over BPD.

A qualified advisor in marginal character problem might be an option for you if you struggle with BPD or feelings. An advisor will have a superior understanding of the roots that lead to your enthusiasm battles. You can both try to control your emotions together.

There are many things you can learn from treatment. You will acquire the necessary skills and responses to address your emotional episodes. You will see a significant improvement in your ability to feel good, which will be beneficial for your everyday relationships and your personal life.

BPD treatment is not the only option. You can also improve your ability and skills to cope with your feelings by using self-help methods.

Autonomic regulation can be influenced by abuse history

Restoratively unexplained medical issues, such as persistent diffuse torment and practical gastrointestinal problems (FGIDs), include intracitating, incapacitating, and expensive. They can be seen over any single medicine setting. Their pathophysiology, however, is not easily understood. Incessant diffuse torment, FGIDs, and other symptoms are becoming more common for those with a history filled with abuse or injury. Patients in torment and gastroenterology facilities will suffer the highest levels of misuse. One examination showed that 67% (of all females) had suffered from sexual or other maltreatment.

Despite the mindfulness, a pathophysiological model that links injury history and misuse history to interminable suffering and FGIDs has a problem. This survey will use the Polyvagal Theory structure. It is a transformative neuroscience model of the autonomic react to health and danger. We draw a pathophysiological device that is established in interminable self-destructive autonomic reactions. It offers ascent to fundamental changes in the direction of agony pathway and the gastrointestinal tract. To give an imaginable model to the starting point of post-awful constant diffuse and unnaturally restorative agony, we use evidence from medication and physiology. This audit does not cover every possible physical problem. It focuses on fibromyalgia, fractious within disorder (IBS), and other clutters due to their wide clinical pervasiveness.

Fibromyalgia (or Fibromyalgia) is a condition that causes pain in muscles, tendons, ligaments and other parts of the body. It is the most widespread form of interminable diffuse pain, with a prevalence rate between 2 and 3 percent. According to research, confusion is more common in women than in men. The number of trademarks affected, their chronicity, as well as the rejection of any other problems that might be causing distress are often factors in determining how to treat it. While the cause of fibromyalgia's symptoms is still unknown, and the pathophysiology of the condition is not clear enough, there is increasing understanding of how passionate or physical injury can trigger or exacerbate side effects.

IBS is a gastrointestinal disorder that presents as continual stomach pain. It can also be characterized by altered inside propensities such as loose bowels and clogging. The current criteria defines peevish inner disorder as repetitive stomach pain, which is generally found in one day of every week for three months. There are two factors that may be more important: (a. connection to stool, (b. relationship with stool change, or (c. relationship with stool structure adjustment (Rome IV criteria). It's the most common gastro-intestinal condition. It represents about 30% all referrals to gastroenterologists. After a meta-examination involving 80 investigations with more than 250,000 subject data, it was found that 11.2% of the total predominance rate is female and higher for men. While the cause and pathophysiology for peevish digestive disorder are still unclear, they do not have fibromyalgia.

We investigate evidence for fibromyalgia. In quest for this, this paper audits: (1) the raised commonness of fibromyalgia and peevish entrail disorder among sexual maltreatment and assault survivors, (2) the sorting out autonomic risk reaction standards drawn from the directing structure of the Polyvagal Theory that clarify the versatile capacity of movements in autonomic state reflected in respiratory sinus arrhythmia (high recurrence pulse fluctuation), (3) the autonomic and neurophysiological frameworks that control torment and gastrointestinal capacity, (4) experimental proof of lessened RSA reflecting adjusted autonomic capacity in fibromyalgia and bad tempered gut disorder patients, (5) regular autonomically-managed co-morbidities in fibromyalgia and crabby gut disorder patients, and (6) proof for autonomic disturbance after injury. The understanding of fibromyalgia/fractious inside disorders as foundational breakness caused by an interminable Autonomic Risk Reaction gives new chances for treatment.

After sexual abuse and rape, Fibromyalgia or Irritable Bowel Symptoms (Fibromyalgia)

This issue covers both youth and old age sexual and physically maltreatment. Based on large-scale meta examinations, 13% of youth sexual maltreatment rates (8% men, 18% women) and 23% of youth physical abuse (19) were found. The Centers for Disease Control and Prevention estimates that assaults occur in lifetimes of 19% for women and 2% for their male counterparts. In the US, cozy accomplice predominance stands at 32% for women and 28% for the men. (With extreme private accomplice cruelty pervasiveness at 22, and 14%, respectively) (20). These higher levels of sexual and bodily maltreatment are also reflected in the prevalence of fibromyalgia (sex-explicit pervasiveness) and fractious bladder disorder (fractious entrail syndrome). Women are nearly twice as likely to have fibromyalgia than men and have 1.67 higher chances of developing bad tempered stomach disorder.

Combining evidence from several investigations across multiple cases shows that misuse history provides a strong indicator for fibromyalgia. Hauser, associates and others found that those who had been subject to physical and sexual abuse in adolescence as well as adulthood predicted more severe fibromyalgia. Paras and Associates found that assault survivors had a particularly high likelihood of developing fibromyalgia from their meta-examination. OR = 3.27. These hazard elements are more prevalent in fibromyalgia victims than in those with chronic rheumatoid inflammation.

The risk of gastrointestinal disorders, such as the peevish-entrail disorder, is also higher in those who have overcome their abuse. Meta-diagnostic data supports this finding that youth sexual mistreatment is linked to a greater risk of developing gastrointestinal issues. It has been shown that people who have experienced sexual maltreatment in their past are twice as likely for gastrointestinal and stomach issues. As seen with fibromyalgia assault survivors are the most vulnerable. Meta-diagnostic tools suggest their likelihood of having a functional gastrointestinal issue is multiple times higher than those without any history of maltreatment. Maltreatment history can lead to more severe GI symptoms and greater need for treatment.

Chapter 12: Vagus Nerve Yoga
A Mind-Body Solution To Well-Being

The vagus is a key component of your physical and mental health. The vagus stretches from your scalp to your stomach. It also enervates you heart and lungs. It also binds your throat muscles and facial muscles. It is possible to have profound effects on the sound of vagus nerves by practicing yoga. Vagus nervous yoga restores balance between body & mind by using mindfulness and deliberate meditation.

"Healthy Vagal Tone can be described as an ideal combination from parasympathetic to sympathetic nervous activity that allows you to react with tolerance and adapt to the ups, downs, and surprises of life. You will find 7 Vagus Nerve Yoga Activities to help you manage tension, improve emotional balance, and more. "Vagus Nerve And Your Wellbeing.

Your nervous systems is built around the tension between two contradicting acts. The sympathetic nervous network is concerned about the fight or run response that occurs due to the production of cortisol. Parasympathetic refers to healing, growth, or recovery. These two sections of your nervous system's autonomic nervous system are meant to work in rhythmic alteration. This is a cycle that promotes healthy periods of alertness as well as restfulness that foster mental and physical health.

Unexplained abuse and chronic stress can lead to a disruption in the harmony between the parasympathetic, supportive and protective roles of your nervous. Our world is too stimulating and triggers our sympathetic nervous system. We all need tools that enable us to activate our parasympathetic nervoussystem on a daily base. The sympathetic nervous function can be inhibited because of the vagus neural. Activities that activate your vagus nerve have a calming affect on your mind and body. Also, it is important to understand that people suffering from untreated PTSD tend to have a predominant parasympathetic nervous systems manifestation that can lead to weakness or depression. If untreated, chronic stress can lead to PTSD and other forms of unexplained mental health problems. Read more about Stephen Porges' Polyvagal hypothesis here. If you are feeling overwhelmed, afraid or trapped, there are activities that can help you to relax the vagus.

A higher vagal tone correlates with decreased inflammation and better prognosis among people with chronic diseases, anxiety, or depression. The intake of food can affect the vagal tone. This is known by Heart Rate Variability (HRV). A good vagal tone involves a slight rise in inhalation heart rates and a drop in exhalation heart rates. It can be thought of as the optimal balance between sympathetic and parasympathetic nervous-system behavior. Higher HRV means that people with greater HRV are able to quickly switch between calm and anticipation. They also have greater ability to heal from stress.

You will learn strategies to control activity of your vagus nervous system. These include changing the speed of your movements, practicing conscious awareness and testing dynamic yoga positions to help you make decisions about activation or excitement. Through somatic consciousness, you might modify your breathing to promote calm alertness. This can help to activate your creativity and allow you to focus on the right things. You can actually learn unique relaxation techniques to help with your evening sleep and relax.

Vagus nerve yoga

The goal of vagus nervous yoga is to be more versatile. Yoga has been proven to be extremely beneficial for stress reduction, improved vagal tone and healing from trauma. This will enable you to shift between a parasympathetic, compassionate, and sympathetic nervous system with greater ease. These seven yoga poses for vagus nerves will help develop a safe and balanced vagal tone.

1. Aware Breathing is key to changing the balance between parasympathetic nerve system behavior and sympathetic. Vagus Nerve Yoga emphasizes diaphragmatic relaxation. It also encourages lengthening of the exhalation. This is to avoid any over

stimulation of the sympathetic nervous systems. Evidence shows that steady, rhythmic, diaphragmatic breathing is beneficial for balancing the vagal tone. Ujjayi pranayama - a type of yogaic breathing that causes mild constriction in your throat and affects your whispering muses - is one example. For this to work, try breathing out of the mouth like you're fogging up your mirror. Instead of doing this, close your eyes and inhale through your nose. You will notice that your wind tone becomes stronger. It often feels almost like the ocean's waves. Start counting your inhalation as well as exhalation. To calm you even further, gradually increase the duration of your exhalation relative it the inhalation. For example, you might start with a 4-count breath and then increase the exhalation length to 6, 8 or 6 counts. This has a relaxing effect in your parasympathetic nervous.

2. Half-Smile. Engaging in a "half smile" can help you change your mental state. It also helps to keep you relaxed. Relaxing your face, turning your mouth slightly and relaxing your neck muscles will increase your vagus nerve's tone. This will activate the "internal neurological network," Dr. Stephen Porges' most advanced branch, the vagus neural. Imagine your smile softening when you smile. You will feel a warm sensation in your mouth and on your neck. Notice the subtle changes in how your thoughts and emotions are consistent.

3. To softly activate the vagus nervous system, open your heart. You can do yoga postures that revolve around your chest and neck. To begin this gentle heartwarming exercise, raise your hands and reach for your arms. Take a deep breath and extend your arms straight across the front. Next, lift your head up by

lifting your elbows. Keep your mouth closed and your elbows straight in front of you. In this movement meditation, take a few deep breathing in. Focusing on the inhalation can calm and lift your mood. Grow into your open-hearted self.

4. Stretch and Wake Up: Yoga can help you to get up in the morning or to feel more awake in the afternoon. Take a look at virabhadrasana, a standing position of a warrior to awaken your mind. Take note of the foot to earth link on staying grounded to energize your body in a balanced way. To stay grounded and connected with the stimuli around you, allow your breath rhythm to keep you breathing steady.

5. Open the Belly. This will allow you to examine the vagus nervous system as it moves through your stomach. With your hands under your arms and feet beneath your thighs, find your way to a sitting position. If you feel pain, place a folded

blanket under you. Keep inhaling and lifting your head up and shoulders. Then, when you enter Cow Pose, lower your belly down to the floor. Exhale as you lower your head to Cat Pose. The timing of your actions should be determined by your heart. As many times as possible to give a soothing treatment to your stomach or back.

6. Self-Compassion or "Loving Kindness" meditation: Self compassion and the practice "loving-kindness" encourage you to love others as well as yourself. Research has shown that loving-kindness meditation can increase vagal tone, improve autonomic range, and produce more positive emotions. Consider the obstacles that you face in daily life. Picture someone else facing the exact same obstacle. How can you make this person feel loved? You can feel this love in your body. You can now send them your best wishes. Let's see

if we can show that same kind of love to ourselves. Okay.

7. Meditation Nidra: This restorative meditation can help calm and slow down the nervous systems. Yoga Nidra (also known as yoga night or calming meditation) is an old method. Yoga Nidra can be an alternative to our hectic modern lifestyle. It allows us to heal our bodies and minds by stimulating the parasympathetic nerve system. To learn more about yourself and your air, you can choose to sit on the floor, on a pillow, or on a yoga mat. Give yourself permission to do whatever you like, even if there is discomfort, heaviness, constriction. To truly calm and care, you should allow yourself to linger at least 30 minutes.

Yoga will help you overcome stress and prevent depression.

Our stress can also be reduced by doing exercises such as meditation, walking, or hiking. We are also subject to scathing comments and questions so often that we start to wonder if they really do mean it. Is this based on sound clinical evidence that exercise is so helpful for people with depression?

There's plenty of research that shows yoga, along with other forms of exercise, can be a great way to manage depression. According to the Department of Health and Human Services' 2008 Overview of the Recommendations in Physical Activity, the report states that there are many studies that show that people who exercise regularly have positive attitudes and less depression symptoms.

You should also be careful when choosing what kind of exercise to do. Different types of exercise are suitable for therapeutic purposes. Some may be more challenging than others. Others might be less demanding. The best way to treat depression is to practice yoga consistently.

Numerous studies have proven that yoga is good for mental health. Some research has shown that yoga improves the blood levels of cortisol. The power of yoga in reducing serotonin levels has been confirmed by a later analysis.

A 2009 study of 54 participants found that they were closely related to one another after and before two weeks of yoga. A total of 64 percent of the participants experienced positive attitude changes. 53 percent also reported decreased symptoms of depression.

An eminent yoga writer has claimed that yoga can help with depression when one's mental focus is turned away from the negativity and towards the benefits of yoga. Meditation breathing exercises can also be used as stress management. These workouts stimulate the vagus nervous, which is believed help to relieve depression symptoms. A particular relaxation technique has been found to result in a 73 percent reverse of major depressions. Other explorations, as well as recommendations from yoga coaches, are compatible with yoga's positive effects on depression and mental outlook. It doesn't matter which strategy you choose, it's what you feel most relaxed with. A yoga therapy expert was looking for someone who can "make you feel as if your life has been transformed" when you leave the yoga studio. And you're energized and full-of-life. Do not change your medications if you are a yoga practitioner. For at least nine months, you should practice daily yoga, regardless of positive results. Only then, can you seriously consider quitting your prescription antidepressants.

See a psychologist immediately to discuss a coach in meditation to help you overcome anxiety and depression. Let yoga get rid of the miseries in your life, now and for ever!

Yoga's benefits - Flight Or Fighting

Yoga can greatly improve your medical condition. Yoga can be used to reduce the adverse effects of conditions such a lung disease or Parkinson's disease. It can also help alleviate joint pain and high blood pressure. Many doctors and yoga teachers accept the benefits of yoga as a viable alternative.

Heat is a leading cause of many illnesses today. According to the Surgeon general, "80%" of all people who die from causes other than trauma actually die from stress disorders. It is no surprise that people look for other solutions in today's fast-paced country.

The practice of yoga can be used as a remedy. It is normal for tension in the brain to increase.

Our nervous system reacts to external discomfort just like it does to other people. Current situations, which are known as "Fight or Flight," have an effect on both our metabolisms and well-being. When we face risk, either real or imagined it is the subconscious that trains the body to take action in one of these circumstances. It manifests in increased heart beat, higher blood pressure, or the shutting off of excessive body functions such digestion. Both mechanisms rely on either "run", or "combat." Breathing becomes slower, muscles contract as they anticipate battle and blood flow to vital parts is restricted. The digestive and removal processes are not working properly. This could be beneficial as the body is prepared to protect itself.

When the situation is more serious, however, it can cause problems. The "flight-or-fight" situation is only intended to be temporary. You can see the negative effects that long-term exposure will have on your body. Yoga may be able to help.

The parasympathetic nervous sistem, or "relaxation instinct", is the counter-measure to "fight or fight". The primary nerves of parasympathetic systems are the vagus or 10th-cranial nerves. They are located within the oblongata, medulla. Parasympathetic activation can cause a slowing down of the pulse, lowering the blood pressure and increased blood supply. This reflex can be caused by yoga. Yoga encourages the pupil's to slow down and relax their muscles. The benefits of practicing yoga are clear. The body responds faster to yoga, and stress's harmful effects are rising.

Yoga is concerned with the idea of reducing stress and improving mindfulness. Yoga offers a way to confront the dilemma of "war/flight", where one must contemplate and then relax the soul. Focusing on practice can help one focus on finding the solution and not on reacting immediately to stimuli. One is able to stay positive and to take care their stressors.

Yoga is a powerful practice. Anyone can achieve the balance and harmony in their lives by practicing this ancient practice. One aspect does not solve all of life's problems. The average person living in the modern world can have a happier, healthier lifestyle by combining meditation with the wonders of modern science as well as ancient curing methods.

Conclusion

Looking at social behavior across life spans, we find significant stretches where self-regulated behaviors, such as spontaneous social engagement, are easily communicated. However, this timetable is held together by a dependence on caregivers. This reliance upon caregiver is coupled with limitations in the neural regulation for autonomic states via the myelinated vigas. Future research is needed to determine if neuropeptides are able to modulate caregiver reliance. Perhaps regulation of oxytocin can be used to allow older and younger children to be more flexible in choosing their caregivers and to have support from a range of caregivers. As neural control circuits increase and social interactions are greater, it is possible that oxytocin/vasopressin can play an even more important role in controlling the state of the brain to help establish solid social bonds.

Humans are social mammals and, as such, they are dependent on other species for survival. When conditions are optimal, this reliance will be both harmoniously and reciprocally. The neural, autonomic and neuroendocrine bases of sociality can be shared with other species. This allows for cross-species comparison of the mechanisms that underpin sociality. Knowledge of the neurobiology underlying social engagement and social hold can give us insight into human ideas. For example, we can learn how social help and caregiving can contribute to good health and recovery after sickness. These systems are integrated through the entire body, including the brainstem. There hormones such oxytocin- and vasopressin have an impact on behavior and the autonomic sense system. Present-day brain structures, such as the cortex, perceive projections from and to these ancient systems as diffuse, but sometimes with ground-breaking sentiments and feelings. The neuroendocrine-autonomic systems that provide high levels in social behavior and social bonds also regulate distressing interactions and the ability for the mammalian to heal itself. The brainstem activities and the autonomic systems have to be subordinate, however. The release oxytocin is able to improve and restore health, in either a situation of safety or an acute stressor that is comparatively mild. In the case of fear or constant pressure, the actions and outcomes of the same adaptive system may be detrimental or fatal. Information about the evolutionary beginning points and neurobiology and sociality of mammals provides a context for understanding both the causes of and the effects of caregiving behaviors

www.ingramcontent.com/pod-product-compliance
Lightning Source LLC
Chambersburg PA
CBHW050408120526
44590CB00015B/1875